*Supporting your Child with Selective Mutism* is accompanied by a number of printable online materials, designed to ensure this resource best supports your professional needs

Go to https://resourcecentre.routledge.com/speechmark and click on the cover of this book

Answer the question prompt using your copy of the book to gain access to the online content.

You can also download more forms, tables, charts at teacherpayteacher.com by searching Junhua Reitman.

# SUPPORTING YOUR CHILD WITH SELECTIVE MUTISM

This book provides strategies and ideas to support children with selective mutism in school, at home, and in the community. Packed with illustrations, this practical guide offers a roadmap to help children overcome selective mutism in various situations.

Based on Junhua Reitman's vast experience of working with her own daughter Amelia – known in the book as Amy, and other children, this book furnishes parents and teachers with a toolkit to plan and implement intervention with individual children throughout their journey from the classic selective mutism 'freeze' response, to talking freely in various settings.

Techniques covered include:

- Graded questioning

- The buddy system

- The rainbow bridge

- Voice exposure

The reader is offered detailed examples of what worked for Amy in a variety of situations, including in school, at breaktimes, in extra-curricular activities, on playdates, and at birthday parties. These examples are followed up with suggestions and ideas of how these experiences could be applied to other children, making it ideal reading for anyone involved in the care of a child with selective mutism.

**Junhua Reitman** is a Parent Coach specialising in counselling parents and teachers of children with selective mutism (SM). She is the co-author of *The Selective Mutism Workbook for Parents and Professionals* and the lead English-to-Chinese translator of several selective mutism related books. She is the director of SunnyMindED Selective Mutism Center. Junhua is also a Montessori early childhood educator.

**Amelia Reitman** is a 16-year-old student in a Biomedical Sciences Academy. Having experienced and overcome selective mutism (SM) as a young child, Amy makes it her personal mission to help children with SM. She is an active volunteer at the Selective Mutism Association and helped with translating and editing books related to SM. Amy works with a group of volunteers to help children with SM make friends and have fun.

**Nianhua Xu** obtained her doctoral training in the field of biomedical sciences and is the co-founder of SunnyMindED. She is a Parent Coach and an active volunteer helping parents of children with selective mutism (SM) on their journey to overcome SM. Nianhua translated several SM-related books into Chinese.

# SUPPORTING YOUR CHILD WITH SELECTIVE MUTISM

## A PRACTICAL GUIDE FOR SCHOOL, HOME, AND IN THE COMMUNITY

Junhua Reitman, Amelia Reitman, and Nianhua Xu

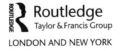

Routledge
Taylor & Francis Group

LONDON AND NEW YORK

First published 2024
by Routledge
4 Park Square, Milton Park, Abingdon, Oxon OX14 4RN

and by Routledge
605 Third Avenue, New York, NY 10158

*Routledge is an imprint of the Taylor & Francis Group, an informa business*

*British Library Cataloguing-in-Publication Data*
A catalogue record for this book is available from the British Library

*Library of Congress Cataloging-in-Publication Data*
Names: Reitman, Junhua, author. | Reitman, Amelia, author. | Xu, Nianhua, author.
Title: Supporting your child with selective mutism : a practical guide for school, home, and in the community / Junhua Reitman, Amelia Reitman, Nianhua Xu.
Description: Abingdon, Oxon ; New York, NY : Routledge, 2024. | Includes bibliographical references. |
Identifiers: LCCN 2023036074 (print) | LCCN 2023036075 (ebook) |
ISBN 9781032409078 (hardback) | ISBN 9781032409085 (paperback) |
ISBN 9781003355267 (ebook)
Subjects: LCSH: Selective mutism—Popular works.
Classification: LCC RJ506.M87 R45 2024 (print) | LCC RJ506.M87 (ebook) |
DDC 618.92/855—dc23/eng/20230824
LC record available at https://lccn.loc.gov/2023036074
LC ebook record available at https://lccn.loc.gov/2023036075

ISBN: 978-1-032-40907-8 (hbk)
ISBN: 978-1-032-40908-5 (pbk)
ISBN: 978-1-003-35526-7 (ebk)

DOI: 10.4324/9781003355267

Typeset in DIN Schriften
by Deanta Global Publishing services Chennai India

Access the Support Material: https://resourcecentre.routledge.com/speechmark

For children on their journey to overcome SM

your courage and bravery are the sources of the change. For parents who are their children's advocates

   your perseverance and creativity drive the changes.

For teachers who support children with SM

   your commitment and extra effort make the child realise their full potential.

For people in the child's life, the classmate, friends, and siblings

   your kindness and acceptance of who they are and always being available make the change possible.

You all are the angels!

Junhua, Amelia, and Nianhua

# CONTENTS

List of Tables — xvi

List of Figures — xvii

List of Forms — xviii

Acknowledgements — xix

Foreword — xx

Preface — xxii

About This Book — xxv

**Part 1   About Selective Mutism — 1**

Preschool Graduation Concert – About SM — 2

The Possible Symptoms of Child with
    Selective Mutism — 4

Challenges in School — 6

The Cycle of Negative Reinforcement — 8

SM Recovery Journey — 9

Supporting Your Child with SM at School,
    Home, and Community
    (The Supporting Triangle) — 11

Talking Five Factors/Talking Formula — 14

The Essential Eight for SM Management — 17

SM Treating Professional – Essential
    Component No. 2 — 20

Contents

SMart Village – Essential Component No. 4    22

Buddy System – Essential Component No. 6    25

**Part 2   Parents Become Advocates
Inside and Outside of School**    **28**

Parents Are the No. 1 Essential
Component in SM Recovery Journey    30

Parents' Dos and Don'ts List    33

Spending Quality Time with Your Child    35

Bringing Pets to the School Playground    37

Child's Participation, the Essential
Component No. 8 – Talk to Amy about
Her SM and Make an Action Plan    39

Reward Calendar    40

Parents Volunteer at School – Cafeteria    47

Parents Volunteer at School – Gardening Club    49

Parents Volunteer at After-school
Club – Girl Scouts    51

Preparing for Going to School in the Morning    53

Riding the School Bus and Bus Buddy    55

Sliding-in    57

Dad Playing Games with Amy in the
Classroom Corner    58

Introduce a New Person into the Game    60

New Person Slides In    62

Parent Slides Out   64

Playing Games in Counsellor's Office   66

Counsellor and Amy Teamed Up   68

Counsellor Practised SM Strategies   70

Amy's Talking Circle Gets Expanded   72

**Part 3   School Staff Providing Support inside and outside of School**   **74**

Letter to Teaching Staff   76

Teachers Are the No. 3 Essential Component in SM Recovery Journey   78

Dos and Don'ts List for Teachers   82

Visiting New School before the New Year/ Term/Semester   84

Back to School Night   86

Private Tour (Left) and Moving up Day (Right) before School Year End   88

Private Time with Counsellor and Buddy   90

Teacher's Home Visit   92

Teacher's Arrival   94

Teacher Participates in Child's Work/Activity   96

Teacher and Child Decorating Cookies Together   98

Rapport Building with Teachers after School and on School Break   100

Contents

Little Broadcaster – Meeting Teacher
    outside of School                    102

Private Time with Teacher/Classmate in the
    School Cafeteria                   104

Painting with Teacher – One-on-One Time in a
    Private Room                     106

Racing Boats – With Teacher and
    Talking Buddy in a Private Room     108

Playing in a Small Group at the
    Classroom Corner                 110

Circle Time/Presentation in Front of
    the Class                       112

One-on-One Time with the Teacher
    between Classes                   114

Communication Book               116

The Task Book                     118

Language Teacher's Helper and Shadow   120

Language – Support from a Shadow Teacher  122

Private Tutor and School Teacher in
    After-School Program for Academic
    and Second Language            124

Academic and After-School Programs,
    Team Sports, Clubs, and Volunteer
    Groups                     126

Maintain Progress during Summer Break  128

## Part 4   Challenges the Child May Face at School 130

Identifying Child's Challenge and
  Providing Support in School                       131

Meet Classmates/Teachers outside of
  School in the Morning                             133

Greet Teachers and Students                         135

Walk to the Building with Classmates/
  Teacher in the Morning                            137

Go to the Bathroom with a Bathroom Buddy            139

School Challenge – Break Time/Recess                141

Butterfly Project 1 – Classroom Observation         143

Butterfly Project 2 – Bring Butterflies to
  School Counsellor's Office                        145

Butterfly Project 3 – Show and Tell                 147

Butterfly Project 4 – Release
  Butterflies into Nature                           149

Subject Helper in Technology Class                  151

Answer Questions in Class with Support              154

Read and Discussion Time in the Library             156

Music Class                                         158

Practice Physical Activities in a Small
  Group before Doing It with Whole Class            160

Ask for Help in Art Class                           162

Science Substitute Teacher                          164

Contents

Take a Test                                                        166

Holiday Party                                                      168

Watch Out for Unhelpful Comments and Bullies      170

Showcase Talent/Skills – Essential
    Component No. 7 in the Recovery
    Journey – Chinese Harp (Guzheng)
    Performance in the Music Class                        172

Picture Day                                                        174

**Part 5   Support for the Child at Home
and in the Community                                     176**

Playdate – Essential Component No. 5 in
    SM Recovery Journey                                     177

Team Sports – After-School Program
    Hosted in School                                           182

Small Animal Club                                             184

Birthday Party 1 – Birthday Party Invitation        186

Birthday Party 2 – Welcome Friends                 188

Birthday Party 3 – Piñata                                    190

Birthday Party 4 – Class Presentation of
    Birthday Party Video                                       192

Negative Thoughts and What Actually
    Happened                                                      194

Playdate at Home – Shopping Role-Play           196

Playdate in Community                                      198

Attending a Birthday Party 200

Go Snow Sledding with Classmates 202

Camping with Classmates and Neighbours 204

Talents and Skills – Play with Neighbours
        in the Community 206

Catch Me If You Can – Fun Time with
        Families and Friends 208

Shopping 1 – Discuss the Shopping
        List before Arriving (Left)
        and Check off the Items on the
        Shopping List (Right) 210

Shopping 2 – Get Help from the
        Clerk without Speaking (Left)
        and Check Out Items and Pay at
        the Cashier (Right) 212

Reading Paws in Township Library 214

Yard Sale and Lemonade Stand
        in the Community 216

**Part 6   Overcoming Selective Mutism and
Gaining Social Skills** **218**

Dance All the Way – Amy Overcomes SM 219

Going Out and Moving Forward – Gaining
        Social Skills through Clubs,
        Volunteering, and Jobs 220

Index 223

# TABLES

| | | |
|---|---|---|
| 1.1 | Eight essential components | 18 |
| 1.2 | SMart Village | 23 |
| 2.1 | Parents the No. 1 essential component in SM recovery journey | 32 |
| 3.1 | Teacher/staff support in the child's SM recovery journey | 79 |
| 3.2 | Tasks and points – Prepare at home and update periodically | 119 |
| 4.1 | Talk openly about anxiety and recognise strength/talent/skills | 132 |
| 5.1 | Playdate five factors facilitating communication | 178 |
| 5.2 | Activity five factors facilitating communication | 179 |

# FIGURES

1.1   Misconceptions about selective mutism versus insights
      from a child with SM                                        5
1.2   The cycle of negative reinforcement                         8
1.3   Communication Stages                                        13
1.4   Buddy system                                                25
2.1   Set up tasks, earn points, redeem rewards and
      achieve goals                                               42
2.2   Small steps lead to destination and big steps
      lead to? (Setbacks)                                         45
2.3   Sliding-in                                                  57
3.1   How to use the task book                                    118

# FORMS

1.1    Anxiety Measurement Hand Chart on a Scale of 1 to 5          16

1.2    SMart Village – Name List of Helper          24

1.3    Buddy System Name List In/ Outside of School          27

2.1a   Communication Steps Tasks, Points, Rewards, and
       Goals Weekly          43

2.1    Communication Steps Tasks, Points, Rewards, and
       Goals Weekly          44

3.1    Tasks Book – Tracking Tasks in School          119

4.1    Teacher's Helper/Subject Helper Work Tracking          153

5.1    Playdate and Progress Tracking          180

5.2    Recording How the Child's Feelings Change before and
       after an Activity          195

# ACKNOWLEDGEMENTS

We sincerely appreciate the incredible efforts of our writing team, illustrators, and volunteers. Your unwavering dedication and boundless encouragement have been the driving force behind making this project a reality. Thank you from the bottom of our hearts for all you have done.

Xuantong (Tom) Wang, Sam Haines Wang, Danielle Wang, Yiqin Cai, XinRu Mai (illustrator), Andrea Reitman, Albert Wang, Richard Wang, Albert Wen, Sophie Wen, and Qi Zha (illustrator), Hannah Diao, and Sabrina Tang.

We want to extend a special note of gratitude to an extraordinary individual whose guidance has been instrumental in helping numerous children with Selective Mutism (SM) embark on their path toward recovery. She shared her extensive expertise and personal experiences in dealing with SM. Her patience, kindness, and willingness to impart her knowledge have impacted our journey. Maggie Johnson, thank you for your remarkable contributions.

# FOREWORD

When I met Mrs. Reitman a few years ago, she was the principal of Stream Montessori School in New Jersey. She shared how Montessori philosophy, pedagogy, and especially teachers help children with selective mutism (SM) and her personal story dealing with SM. I recognised her achievements and was amazed by the efforts of the parents and teachers who worked together to help her daughter overcome SM. Her mission to help children with SM and their families is admirable. Earlier, she co-authored *The Selective Mutism Workbook for Parents and Professionals* with Maggie Johnson. And now, she has taken the time to publish this book for parents and teachers.

In my experience as a teacher and principal, I observed that teachers and supportive parents achieved the best results in opening the channel of communication of a child with SM. This is not easy, and the results come from intentional actions. Most SM children are intelligent, kind, and quiet in class. They often have difficulty telling the teacher when they have challenges with classwork or peers. Children with SM are less demanding than others and generally do not attract attention from the teachers. However, they need more intentional preparation for the environment to begin their connection with the world.

Teachers are often the first to observe and identify irregular student behaviour. Usually, their experiences with children allow them to identify differences and deviations in developmental markers much earlier than the child's parents. The early diagnosis and intervention reduce the recovery period and the child's suffering of being silent and increase the family's happiness. However, only some teachers have experience and training in supporting the child with SM. As a result, the SM child may be misdiagnosed as a quiet, observant child.

Children with SM bring curiosity and eagerness to explore just as other children do. However, the silence and stiffness from the anxiety about their environment often make them hesitant to express themselves and connect with others. Even so, SM children can feel safe, take calculated risks, ask questions, make mistakes, learn to trust, and share their feelings with the full support of their teachers, parents, and buddies.

This guide includes theoretical insights based on personal and professional experience with SM children and parents. Demonstrating multiple strategies in various situations helps caregivers, teachers, and classmates build communication with children with SM.

In addition, the book provides SM knowledge through stories, pictorial examples, and practical ways to offer advice through observation and identification that help SM children conquer anxieties and relate to their community. Readers will learn best practices that encourage a child with critical life messages coming through, by word or action, such as I believe in you, I trust you, I know you can do this, you are safe, and you are important to me.

Enjoy your journey of opening the door of communication to an SM child.

Regards,
*Marsha Stencel, Montessori Educator*

# PREFACE

Six years ago, my daughter Amelia overcame selective mutism (SM) after a few years on the journey. I thought I could finally wash my hands of anything related to SM. Alas, it was not meant to be.

I shared personal stories online about helping my daughter deal with SM, and these stories had legs of their own. Parents of children with SM from many corners of the world reached out to me; they were touched by my stories and wanted to learn how to help their own children.

With a team of dedicated volunteers, I have translated several books about SM from English to Chinese, including *The Selective Mutism Resource Manual* 2nd Ed (SMRM2e) by Maggie Johnson and Alison Wintgens. I also co-authored a book with Maggie, *The Selective Mutism Workbook for Parents and Professionals: Small Steps, Big Changes* (Workbook). I am now a SM coach specialising in helping parents and teachers of children with SM, empowering them to be their children's advocates.

Looking back, I see the bricks of this path have been laid by many kind people: teachers, treating professionals, friends, families, neighbours, volunteers, children with SM and their parents, and kind strangers. Would I want to quit walking down this path? No, not when there are still children struggling to let their voices be heard, not when there are still parents trying to help their beloved children speak up and realise their full potential.

What you are reading now is a selection of carefully chosen strategies and activities that were proven effective in helping children deal with challenges in various situations and overcome their SM. Some of these strategies draw from my personal experience helping my daughter Amy overcome her SM and my experience as a parent coach supporting SM parent groups, helping parents, teachers, and their children deal with challenges in their lives. Others are based on the experiences of working with Ruth Perednick and other professionals.

You will see the influence of Maggie Johnson's work throughout the book, such as her advice with regard to graded questioning, talking via friends and family, whispering, and sliding-in.

As a parent of a child with SM, I used to waste precious time waiting for the "perfect" opportunity to ask a teacher for help, to arrange for a playdate, or to set up a support plan at school. Now I know there is never a perfect time to do the perfect things. I encourage you to use this book as a nudge to take immediate action to work with the school, the SM treating professionals, and your child. After each success, do not sit back and wait for something else to happen. Instead, use the child's progress as a guide to keep moving forward.

Are you a parent or teacher who wants to help a beloved child with SM? Are you that special child yourself? We welcome you to join us on our magical path.

*Junhua Reitman*

***

In the process of SM research and case studies, I was introduced to a group of hundreds or so parents whose children are suffering from SM, a rare and severe form of childhood anxiety disorder, which is also poorly understood in modern society. Many professionals and parents believe that these children are still young and will talk eventually when they get older. Or they confuse a child's silence with shyness or even think it is a personality and does not require any treatment. Some parents may anxiously force their children with SM to talk, unwantedly leading to increased nervousness and anxiety, thus, unable to speak. SM needs to be treated as early as possible. Parents should start taking action immediately to help their children with SM through a series of evidence-based interventions and treatments to reduce their anxiety and guide them to improve their SM condition, so they can break their silence sooner.

*Supporting Your Child With Selective Mutism: A Practical Guide for School, Home, and in the Community* covers the period from kindergarten to elementary school (age 5–10), including knowledge sections and story sections. This Guide intends to disseminate the knowledge of SM to a broader audience and raise awareness of this childhood anxiety. Each story has three parts: illustration, accompanying narrative, and tips and tricks. The stories revolve around the challenges children face at school, focusing on how parents and teachers can create a buddy system to help children with SM navigate challenges inside and outside of school. Through the collection of the stories, we hope readers can grasp how to apply strategies in different situations and adapt them to suit their own concerns to create a supportive environment for children with SM and help them break free from the chain of SM. Together, let's support children with SM to find their confident voices and live healthy, happy, and blissful childhood.

*Nianhua Xu*

***

I had SM for seven years, starting at the age of three. During that time, I only spoke to my parents and brother. My family and friends all loved me dearly, but I could not speak to them at all. I used to struggle in nearly every aspect of school. Preschool and elementary school should be a fun part of life, but I was unable to enjoy it.

Now, I am a 16-year-old student in a Biomedical Sciences Academy. I am still friends with many of my earliest talking buddies who were by my side when I faced difficult talking situations in elementary school. I have been dancing for nine years and now do so competitively. I am a stage manager for the stage crew at my school and enjoy participating in other community events through my involvement in school service and academic clubs. I am passionate about helping others, which has led me to become a volunteer for my local emergency medical services squad.

Meeting new people is no longer challenging for me, and I cannot believe how far I have come. My advice for those who are still trying to overcome SM is to join clubs, teams, programs, and camps where you can meet and get to know others. It is important to find a friend; there will always be someone out there willing to be your friend; you just have to find them, even if it may be scary. Try your best and keep trying; you will see the light at the end of the tunnel eventually.

*Amelia (Amy) Reitman*

# ABOUT THIS BOOK

School is the main focus of Amy's recovery journey because it is where she faces most of her challenges caused by SM. In the book, we share how we tackled each of Amy's challenges using graded exposures and small steps in order to help her gradually face and overcome her fear of speaking. We helped Amy set up a buddy system that consisted of her classmates and friends, and that began her support at home and in the community with help from her family, therapist, buddies, and teachers. Once Amy feels comfortable talking to these people outside of school, we then discuss bringing her support back to school and consider her recovery journey there. For example, with careful planning and execution, Amy starts to let her voice be heard in school by ONE teacher and ONE of her talking buddy classmates in a private room, then moves on to do so in a quiet classroom corner, and eventually, in time, she is able to speak in front of all teachers and students in the classroom, and ultimately talk to anybody anywhere in the school. A variety of strategies are demonstrated by Amy and her supporters.

## How to Use the Guide Effectively

The main goal of the Guide is to empower parents and teachers to become advocates for children with SM. Parents and teachers are encouraged to:

1. Command the SM basics by reading books, watching videos, and joining parent support groups related to SM. *The Selective Mutism Resource Manual 2nd ED* (SMRM2e) and *The Selective Mutism Workbook for Parents and Professionals: Small Steps, Big Changes* (SM Workbook) are excellent resources. We encourage you to tap into these two books for a wealth of information about the whys, whats, and hows. Seek SM treating professional's guidance whenever possible but do not be disheartened if this cannot be arranged. There are many success stories where professionals were not involved.

2. Learn child development knowledge, enhance parenting skills, and, where possible, spend quality time with the child, improve parent–children relationships. Know your child as a unique individual, not just someone with SM. Explore your child's interests and talents instead of focusing on his/her condition. Help your

child transform into a confident and expressive human being. Be positive, be patient, and be creative!

3. Use this Guide as a launch pad rather than a script. Let Amy's story inspire your own creativity and resourcefulness. Not all SM children have the same temperament, enjoyment of competition, and skills or are the same age, so parents should choose the strategies that fit their child the best. Similarly, much of this book draws on Amy's own experience and not all schools or groups will be able to facilitate in the same way. These are however ideas and suggestions that could be experimented with and adapted, in your own settings.

4. You can download more forms, tables, charts at teacherpayteacher.com by searching Junhua Reitman.

# Part 1

# ABOUT SELECTIVE MUTISM

This section provides valuable information and tools for parents and teachers seeking to support children with selective mutism (SM) on their journey to recovery. It begins by describing the possible symptoms of a child with SM and how negative reinforcement can exacerbate these symptoms. It includes a figure that contrasts comments from people who do not understand SM with what the child may express about their condition.

The section provides practical guidance on supporting children with SM in various settings, such as school, home, and the community, and helping the child make connections and transitions among these settings. This guidance includes a figure that outlines the communication steps from nonverbal to verbal, a talking formula that considers five factors that impact talking, and eight essential components that are influential in the child's recovery. Furthermore, in this section, the authors explain the important roles of three out of eight components, namely, treating professionals, a buddy system, and a supportive community. Parents are emphasised as the Number One essential component and the driving force of the child's recovery.

Without waiting for the official diagnosis by SM treating professionals, parents can start to work with the school to help the child overcome SM. The section also includes helpful tables and forms, such as the anxiety measurement hand chart, SMart village form, and a buddy system name list, that parents and teachers can use to implement these essential components.

By the end of this section, readers will have a clear understanding of the challenges children with SM face in school and the importance of intervention strategies in supporting their recovery. This section lays the foundation for the practical examples and strategies in the following sections. Parts 2 and 3 are specifically tailored for parents and teachers, respectively, while Parts 4, 5, and 6 focus on the child.

It should be clarified that this guide is based on the author's own experience with her daughter, and from working with other families with SM. Not all intervention strategies are included in this guide for practical reasons. The authors discuss some of the most fundamental strategies, and when used repeatedly, they can yield remarkable results.

DOI: 10.4324/9781003355267-1

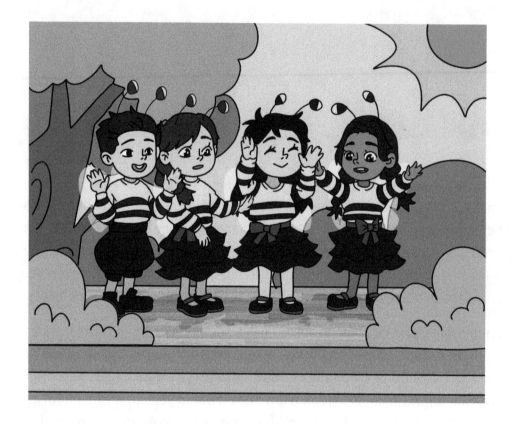

## Preschool Graduation Concert – About SM

It was showtime! Amy had been looking forward to performing on stage for her graduation concert. She had rehearsed the lyrics and moves many times at home. But when the music started, Amy looked like a deer caught in the headlights, frozen and unable to sing or dance like her classmates.

Amy had a condition called selective mutism (SM), an anxiety disorder that caused Amy to become mute in front of certain people and in certain situations. Apart from SM, Amy was a typical girl who was a chatterbox at home with a great sense of humour. She was good at maths and dancing. People who loved Amy and knew her true character called her "SMart Amy".

SM can profoundly affect a child's life, leading to academic, social, emotional, and psychological issues. Preschools and schools are where SM children face most of their difficulties. In addition to not talking in school, other real-life challenges include using the school bathroom, drinking water, having lunch, reporting injuries, etc. SM children may have trouble asking or answering questions in class. They may skip schoolwork, homework, or projects for fear of presenting in front of the class. They may also be afraid to sing in music class or run in P.E. Some children may avoid school altogether. It can be hard for SM children to make friends, maintain relationships, and participate in group activities. If ignored and left untreated, all these issues could turn into further emotional and psychological problems.

## Tips and Tricks

- Educate yourself and educate others about SM. It is a common misunderstanding that SM children choose not to talk. In fact, SM is a phobia, i.e., fear of speaking. It is not a choice and requires intervention.
- Parents, teachers, and therapists working together as a team is the most effective way to help children overcome their SM.

# The Possible Symptoms of a Child with Selective Mutism

**Physical/Health**

1. Shutting down or freezing
2. Awkward body language
3. Lack of eye contact when feeling anxious about the need to talk
4. Skin picking or other repetitive behaviours
5. Pains: Headaches, stomach ache, feeling sick or other pains, particularly before specific activities or events
6. Embarrassment when eating in front of others: not eating in the school cafeteria, being a picky eater
7. Embarrassed to use a public bathroom: has accidents when in public
8. Bedwetting and urinary tract infections from withholding urine
9. Difficulty sleeping/lack of sleep
10. Restlessness

**Social Communication and Personality**

1. Low self-esteem
2. Uncomfortable when introduced to new people
3. Needing constant reassurance
4. Easily frustrated; emotional over "small things"
5. Stubborn, aggressive, assertiveness
6. Mood swings
7. Avoidance, hiding, running away when anxious
8. Negativity
9. Overthinking, difficulty in making choices
10. Intolerance of uncertainty

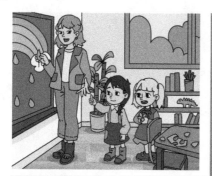
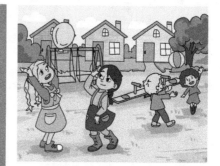
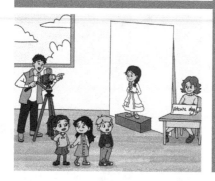
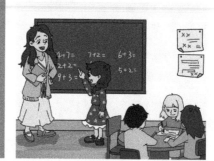

**Sensitivity**

1. Touch (hair brushing, tags, socks)
2. Does not like to be hugged
3. Sound
4. Light
5. Food: taste/textures
6. Smell

**Parents**

1. Anger when questioned by a parent
2. Having meltdowns when getting home from school
3. Asking many questions to allay anxiety

**Academics and School**

1. Perfectionist (fear of making mistakes)
2. Have high expectations for self, including schoolwork & sports
3. Slow at finishing homework
4. Does not do classwork at school
5. Easily frustrated by schoolwork
6. Have more difficulty answering open-ended questions
7. Avoid social activities or events (including school)
8. Anxious when being photographed
9. Dislike of corrections/reminders
10. Difficulty concentrating/Lack of focus

**Comments from People When They Do Not Know about SM**

"I know you can talk. You choose not to talk."

"You don't have to be shy around me."

"Just talk. You have to try."

"Don't ask her. She's weird."

"I can't help if you don't tell me what's wrong."

"You need to join the class activities."

"Speak up. I can't hear you!"

"Look at me while I am talking to you."

"Ask for help if you don't understand."

**What I SAY about Me and SM…**

"I am not shy or rude. I have selective mutism. It is not my choice to not talk."

"SM is an anxiety disorder that prevents me from speaking in certain situations and to certain people. I am smart and I want to talk but words don't come out."

"Do not make a big deal if I talk to you or talk in the classroom."

"Stop pressing me to speak. You make my life harder."

"Give me 5 seconds. I might be able to speak."

"I am too anxious to get the words out. As such, I have trouble participating in group activities verbally. But please invite and include me in your group."

"Sit next to me and play with me."

"I am chatty and can talk freely with my family at home. But I cannot speak when I am out of my comfort zone."

"I may not respond to your questions, but I really want to. With your help, I might be able to do so soon."

**FIGURE 1.1 Misconceptions about selective mutism versus insights from a child with SM**

# Challenges in School

Children with SM do not usually have additional learning challenges. Some may even have above-average grades. Nonetheless, SM may still impact their school performance and other aspects of their life.

*School and Life Challenges*

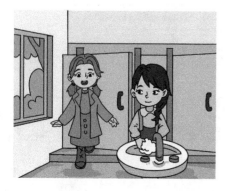

- Using the restroom, drinking water, and eating lunch
- Reporting an injury, stomach pain, physical discomfort, and so on
- Sitting down/getting up/walking around in the classroom

*Academic Challenges*

- Going to school and joining others in the classroom
- Completing classwork at school
- Submitting homework
- Asking questions or seeking clarification in class
- Self-expression in writing
- Oral reading and presentation assignment
- Exercising in PE class or singing in music class

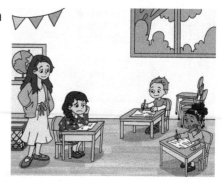

*Social Interaction Challenges*

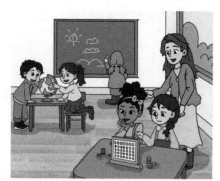

- Initiating conversations or actions
- Participation in group or whole class activities
- Developing and maintaining friendships and interactions with others

## Tips and Tricks

**Teachers may see:**

1. A child who is frozen or zoned-out, unable to do any classwork or participate in any activity that involves language, communication, or movement.
2. A child who is quiet and well-behaved in a structured classroom.

**When teachers do not see or believe that the child has any problems in school:**

1. Child's stress and anxiety build up throughout the day. When the child gets home, they are exhausted and may have a meltdown.
2. Child is unable to let parents know the real situation. They may not understand what is happening to them and be unable to put their teacher's attitude or expectations into words. Or, they may be worried about what teachers have said to them and afraid their parents will think they have been naughty. Often they say everything is good in order to avoid longer conversations with parents and more pressure to speak. They may even deny that they have spoken at school because they are worried this will lead to a greater expectation to talk.
3. Child brings unfinished classwork home. This plus homework will make the child feel overwhelmed.

**What teachers can do when there is a child with SM symptoms in the classroom:**

1. Observe and record/video the child's behaviour if the child has been not talking in certain situations for more than two months.
2. Explain the child's pattern of behaviour at school to parents and seek their help to understand it. Acknowledge that parents know how to bring out the best in their children and ask parents to share a video that shows the child talking with the family at home.
3. Once confirmed that the child's behaviour at home and school are different, parents, teachers, and SM treating professionals should work together to formulate and execute an intervention plan to help the child overcome their SM.

## The Cycle of Negative Reinforcement[1,2]

Negative reinforcement is the key maintaining factor of SM (making the child feel better by removing anxiety, rather than helping them face and overcome their anxiety). When a child is asked a question or prompted to speak, they might feel anxious, zone out, look to their parent, talking buddy, or others (rescuer), and/or not respond. The rescuer might feel distressed knowing the child will not utter a word. To escape this awkwardness, the rescuer may jump in to "rescue" the child by speaking in the child's place. This further reinforces the child's behaviour of not talking. It is crucial to break this cycle of negative reinforcement in order to help the child find their own voice.

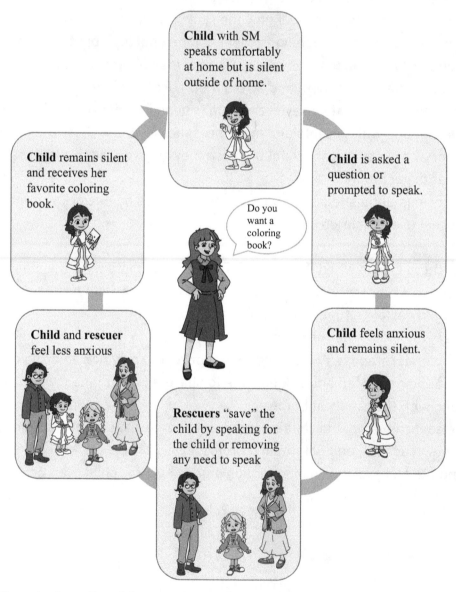

**FIGURE 1.2** The cycle of negative reinforcement

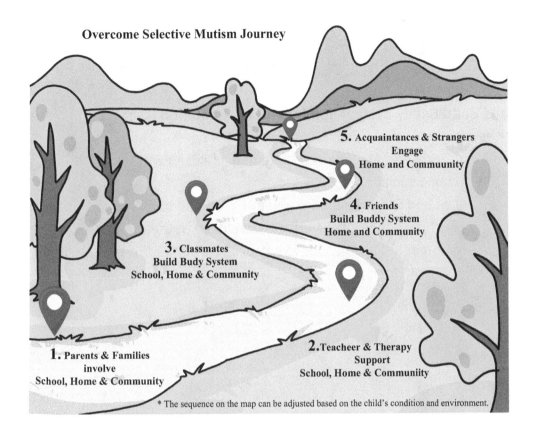

**Overcome Selective Mutism Journey**

5. Acquaintances & Strangers
Engage
Home and Commuunity

4. Friends
Build Buddy System
Home and Community

3. Classmates
Build Budy System
School, Home & Community

1. Parents & Families
involve
School, Home & Community

2. Teacheer & Therapy
Support
School, Home & Communiity

* The sequence on the map can be adjusted based on the child's condition and environment.

## SM Recovery Journey

If overcoming SM is considered a journey, parents, teachers, therapists, classmates, friends, acquaintances, and even strangers are all important participants along the way.

1. **Parents and Families' Involvement in School, Home, and Community:** Parents and families are the best advocates for children with SM. They work closely with teachers and therapists to set goals, formulate a plan, track progress, and, if they choose to, can develop an incentive system where the child has enjoyable activities after achieving goals. They are the liaison between the home/community and the school.

2. **Teachers and Therapist's Support in School, Home, and Community:** Teachers can identify specific areas in which children with SM need help in school. A qualified SM therapist can design an effective intervention plan tailored to individual needs and situations. For further help, tap into resources that the ...ol can provide.

   ...nates Build Buddy System in School, Home, and Community: Classmates ... main force in a buddy system. They can be potential and accompanying buddies at first. Through playdates at home/in public or by attending the same after-school program, classmates become talking buddies of the child with SM. They serve as a bridge to bring a child's voice from home to school and community.

4. **Friends Build Buddy System at Home and Community:** Friends can be children's relatives, neighbours, family friends, children of parents' friends/coworkers, nanny, tutors, coaches etc. These people help children with SM develop social skills and expand social circles.

5. **Acquaintances and Strangers Engaged at Home and in the Community:** Everyone in the life of a child with SM can help at some point in the journey, e.g., a waitress at a restaurant the family dines in weekly or a cashier at the store that the family often visits.

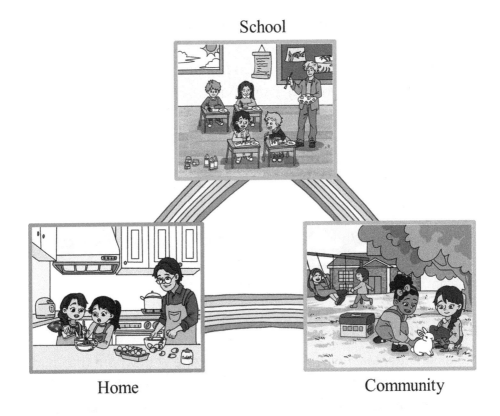

School

Home

Community

## Supporting Your Child with SM at School, Home, and Community (The Supporting Triangle)

To children with SM, school is where they face most of their challenges daily. Some of these challenges are more urgent and require immediate alleviation to maintain a normal and healthy life, e.g., going to the school bathroom and having lunch in the school cafeteria.

There are simple yet effective ways to help SM children in school. Building a buddy system is one of them.

### *The Buddy System*

Depending on the child's specific needs, a teacher can assign an accompanying buddy to sit next to the child and assist him/her when needed. They can pair the child with his/her buddies in the same group for all class activities and group projects. Once the child talks confidently with the buddy sitting next to her/him or in the same group, the teacher can rotate the buddy out and rotate a NEW classmate in.

Next, extend the school buddy system outside of school to home and community. Parents can ask for a class roster from the teacher if one is not readily available.

Based on the child's preference of whom to invite first, parents arrange playdates either at home or in the community. Playdates at home are usually more effective. However, playdates outside the home, such as in a park or a zoo, also work if inviting classmates home is more challenging to arrange. The playdates should be fun and suitable for both parties. Parents should facilitate these playdates to make them effective (see page 177). Other options for meeting classmates outside of school include going on a trip, camping, attending the same club or after-school program, etc. They provide opportunities for the child to build rapport and let his/her voice be heard.

Once the child speaks to his/her classmates outside of school, these classmates become his/her talking buddies. Talking buddies can serve as a bridge to bring the child's voice from outside of school into school.

## The Rainbow Bridge

We think of classmates, teachers, parents, and anyone with whom the child talks as the people on the rainbow bridge connecting the child's world from outside to inside the school. Different people can help, and each person has the uniqueness to help. The more people on the rainbow bridge connecting school, home, and the community, the quicker the child will hopefully overcome SM.

**Communication Five Stages from Nonverbal to Verbal**

The child starts by doing something manageable and is then given the opportunity to do a little more each time. With the proper support, the child may overcome SM, even though they may progress (green arrow), regress (red arrow) or stay the same in their journey. Parents and teachers should understand SM, observe the child's behavior and provide appropriate support, such as assigning a talking buddy to sit next to the child, setting aside **one-on-one** time with the child, providing opportunities to talk rather than demands, or promoting self-esteem by assigning responsibilities such as being a teacher helper or subject helper. Children may whisper or speak quietly initially, but will naturally speak louder as they repeat activities and feel more comfortable.

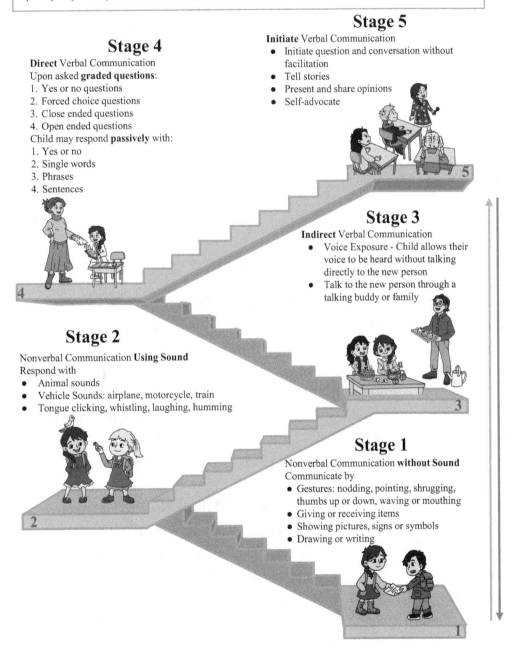

## Stage 5

**Initiate** Verbal Communication
- Initiate question and conversation without facilitation
- Tell stories
- Present and share opinions
- Self-advocate

## Stage 4

**Direct** Verbal Communication
Upon asked **graded questions**:
1. Yes or no questions
2. Forced choice questions
3. Close ended questions
4. Open ended questions
Child may respond **passively** with:
1. Yes or no
2. Single words
3. Phrases
4. Sentences

## Stage 3

**Indirect** Verbal Communication
- Voice Exposure - Child allows their voice to be heard without talking directly to the new person
- Talk to the new person through a talking buddy or family

## Stage 2

Nonverbal Communication **Using Sound**
Respond with
- Animal sounds
- Vehicle Sounds: airplane, motorcycle, train
- Tongue clicking, whistling, laughing, humming

## Stage 1

Nonverbal Communication **without Sound**
Communicate by
- Gestures: nodding, pointing, shrugging, thumbs up or down, waving or mouthing
- Giving or receiving items
- Showing pictures, signs or symbols
- Drawing or writing

**FIGURE 1.3 Communication Stages**

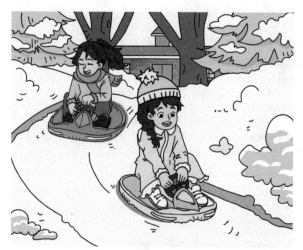
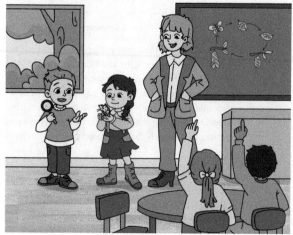

## Talking Five Factors/Talking Formula

Compare the above two situations: on the left was Amy riding a snow slide with her talking buddy Cate at the playground; on the right was Amy doing a show and tell with her talking buddy David in front of the whole class. Guess which situation made it easier for Amy to talk?

Below are five main factors to consider when helping a child with SM speak:

1. **Who to interact with and how many people:** inform the child beforehand whom they will meet and how many people they will interact with, e.g., the number of relatives at a family gathering and who they are.
2. **What activity:** Explain to the child in advance the kind of activity they will participate in. Choose activities that are fun and engaging for the child. Consider the following and choose according to the child's capacity: language, movement, competition, teamwork, and fun.
3. **Where:** Tell the child where the activity takes place, whether it is at home, in school, or somewhere in the community.
4. **Situation:** Let the child know what to expect in different situations, environments, or times of day that they will be involved in, e.g., hanging out with friends in the park, finding a seat during lunch time, performing in a choir after school.
5. **Anxiety level is affected by the above four factors:** Observe the child's body language, eye contact, and facial expression as the less movement the child displays, the more anxious they feel. Knowing the anxiety level helps the adult make sensible adjustments to strategy, activity, and goal.

## Notes

1 Cotter, A., Todd, M. & Brestan-Knight, E. (2018). Parent-child interaction therapy for children with selective mutism (PCIT-SM), Handbook for parent-child interaction therapy, Springer Nature Swizerland AG: 113-128, https://doi.org/10.1007/978-3-319-97698-3_8

2 Kurtz, S. (2016). In focus: Selective Mutism: who put the "C" in the CBT? *In Balance* 31 (1): 10-11, https://www.kurtzpsychology.com/wp-content/uploads/2019/07/SM_Who-Put-the-C-in-the-CBT_In-Balance_Spring-2016.pdf

### Tips and Tricks

- You probably have guessed by now that it was easier for Amy to speak to Cate than to speak in front of the whole class because of the different talking factors involved. These five talking factors impact whether a child speaks or not. Thus, changing one of those factors at a time is essential to keep the talking momentum going.
- Let the child express their anxiety in ways that do not require talking; ask the child to point to an anxiety measurement hand (chart) on a scale of 1–5 to identify their anxiety level.

# Form 1.1 Anxiety Measurement Hand Chart on a Scale of 1 to 5

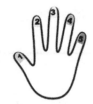

Use this form before participating in activities that cause the child distress, e.g., going to school.

## Before

- Fill out Who, What, Where, Situation, and Anxiety level.
- Explain that 1 is the least anxious and 5 is the most anxious. Ask the child to point out which finger matches their anxiety level.

## After

- Discuss whether the anxiety level is different than expected afterwards and fill out the Improvement section.
- Keep the forms in a binder and use them to remind and acknowledge how much the child has achieved.

| Date | Who | What | Where | Situation | Anxiety level | What actions can improve the situation |
|------|-----|------|-------|-----------|---------------|----------------------------------------|
|  |  |  |  |  | 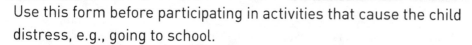 |  |
|  |  |  |  |  |  |  |
|  |  |  |  |  |  |  |
|  |  |  |  |  |  |  |
|  |  |  |  |  |  |  |

## The Essential Eight for SM Management

Eight essential components for managing Selective Mutism (SM) are summarised in Table 1.1. Further information on each element can be found in the corresponding parts shown in column 2.

Components No. 1 to No. 3 highlight the importance of the SM management team, also referred to as the Essential Management Trio. Parents, SM treating professionals, and teachers must work together to implement effective intervention plans and provide essential support to the child on their journey to recovery.

Components No. 4 to No. 8 outline practical actions parents can take once their child is diagnosed with SM. After learning more about SM, the first step is to create a name list of people in the child's environment who can help and start building a support system, referred to as the SMart village (No. 4).

Parents can then arrange playdates (No. 5) with people on the name list one by one, gradually establishing a buddy system (No. 6) that provides the child with a network of supportive friends. Part 5 of the guide focuses on playdates as an effective way to turn names on a list into a support buddy system. These buddies can help the child in school.

Essentials No. 7 and No. 8 are about the child with SM. It is crucial to identify the child's talents and skills (No. 7) and provide opportunities for them to communicate and gain confidence. The child's participation (No. 8) is vital to the success of the intervention plan, and without their cooperation, the plan is just a plan on paper, no matter how well-designed it is.

**TABLE 1.1 Eight essential components**

| Esse. no. | Component | Examples | | |
|---|---|---|---|---|
| 1 | **Parents' support** Initiate work related to school, home, and community. Work with SM treating professionals and teachers to set up intervention plans both in and, where possible, outside of school. Track the progress, revisit and revise the plan (See Part 2) | If the school allows, parents go to the classroom to help the child build rapport with teachers and classmates one by one in the morning, during break time/ recess, lunchtime, after school, or during summer break | Where possible, parents volunteer in the cafeteria and clubs in school, join Parent Teacher Association (PTA), or become classroom parents | Parents educate selves about SM and train and share SM knowledge with teachers and counsellors. Parents can be the key worker who accelerate the child's intervention progress |
| 2 | **SM Treating Professionals' support** SM Diagnosis and train parents and teachers about SM; work with parents and the school to set up the intervention plans (See Part 1, 3) | Therapist meets parents, child, and teacher in their office and school. Talking to the therapist is not enough; the child needs to practise/talk in real-life situations | Where possible the child works one-on-one with the counsellor or speech therapist and special education teacher | Coach other teachers and staff about SM strategies and activities, so they can carry them out with the child's classmates |
| 3 | **Teachers' support** inside and (if possible) outside of the school (See Part 3 and 4) | One-on-one with a teacher and talking buddy in the teacher's office while playing a video of the child's playdate activities (voice exposure) | Home visit-teacher slides in to participate in an activity. The child talks to their talking buddy and parent before the teacher comes, then later in front of the teacher. The activity is fun and engaging for the child | The teacher communicates with the child during the holidays, where possible, to build rapport. When school starts, the teacher and the child will have common topics for interaction |

(Continued)

**TABLE 1.1 (Continued)**

| Esse. no. | Component | Examples | | |
|---|---|---|---|---|
| 4 | **SMart Village** includes everyone who is in the child's life (See Part 1) | Family, friends, and neighbours | School staff, aid, shadow teacher and tutor, playground/lunchtime staff, bus driver, etc. | Strangers, such as clerks, cashiers, waiter/waitress |
| 5 | **Playdates**<br>• With classmates, friends, and their friends<br>• Invite them in and go out to join their activities<br>• The activities should be fun for both sides<br>• Playdate five factors (See Part 5) | Playdate at home: hide and seek, games, cooking, experiment, reading books, call/facetime | Meet classmates in the school playground to build rapport and help parents set up future playdates | Small activities, or bigger ones like going camping and making s'mores with classmates and neighbours |
| 6 | **Buddy system**<br>• School<br>• Outside of school<br>• Talking buddies in and outside of school are the ones on the bridge to connect the child to others (See Part 1) | Utilise a buddy system for going to the bathroom, eating lunch, submitting homework, etc. | Build rapport with teachers and classmates during one-on-one time | Attend activities and programs to foster friendships with classmates and friends |
| 7 | **Showcase talents/skills** Ensure success by setting manageable tasks and considering the child's SM, ability, personality, interest, and hobby (See Part 4, 5) | Seek opportunities to share the child's interests and show their skills in school | Observe chrysalis with accompanying buddies in the teacher's office | Bike, swim, dance, and play sports with a neighbour |
| 8 | **Child participation** Ensure the child is included and adapts to activities so they can participate despite their SM. Parenting skills and relationships with the child play an important role, such as spending quality time, playing games together, and sharing daily experiences (See Part 2, 3, 4, 5) | Educate the child and talk openly to them about their difficulty talking; set goals and tasks. If appropriate for your child, earn points and redeem rewards together | Help the counsellor distribute the event flyer at the school entrance | Have fun and build rapport with supporters (shadow teacher, tutor, nanny, coach) |

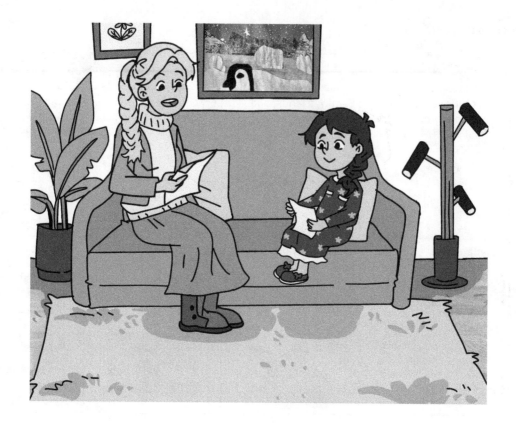

## SM Treating Professional – Essential Component No. 2

Parents play a crucial role in driving the recovery process for children with SM. Therefore, they are considered the top essential component, and Part 2 is specifically dedicated to providing parents with guidance on what can be done and how to do it.

The second essential component is SM Treating Professionals (SMTP). An accurate diagnosis is the first step in the intervention process, and SMTPs are responsible for this task. The ideal intervention cycle involves collaboration between parents, teachers, and SMTPs in treating SM, as depicted in the following diagram.

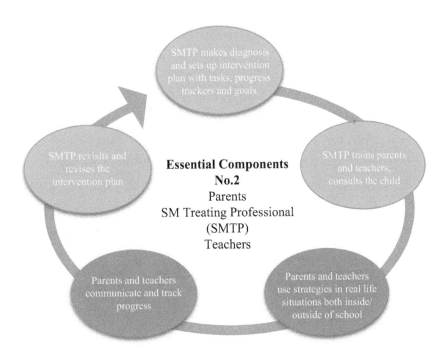

The SM treating professional makes the formal diagnosis, sets up and revises the intervention plan, and educates others. When an SMTP is not accessible, it can be a lay diagnosis: when a child consistently can't speak in certain situations but can speak fine in others, it is much more likely to be SM than shyness. While searching for professionals, parents and teachers can hopefully agree to work together to help the child deal with their difficulties, leading to success stories.

## SMart Village – Essential Component No. 4

It takes a village to raise a child with SM.

Raising a child with SM can be challenging, and it often takes a community to provide the necessary support. Parents can leverage their efforts by working with different groups of people from home, school, and the community. The first step is to create a name list, using Form 1.2 as a guide for identifying the five groups of people who may be able to provide support. Parents should start with family and neighbours that the child is familiar with and comfortable talking to and work their way down to incorporate even strangers in the community. It is important to keep in mind the 4W and 1H – Who to interact with, What activity, What location, When to do the activity, and How to use the strategies. To help with organising thoughts, parents can use Form 1.3, which is also helpful in planning playdates (Essential No. 5. See more in part 5) and activities. Parents can make notes on the form if a person may become the child's buddy. By working with these different groups and utilising these tools, parents can build a supportive Smart Village for their child with SM.

**TABLE 1.2 SMart Village**

| No. | Who can help | What activities help child with SM | | |
|---|---|---|---|---|
| 1 | Parents, families and neighbours' involvement in school, home, and community | Parents, siblings, cousins, relatives | Classmates, schoolmates | Neighbours and friends |
| 2 | Teachers and treating professionals' support in school, home, and community | One-on-one/small group time with the counsellor in a private space | Teacher builds rapport during the breaks | Shadow teacher, tutor, nanny, and coach |
| 3 | Classmates build Buddy System at school, home, and community via after-school programs and playdates | Attend summer camp with classmates in school | Join a small animal club with siblings and classmates | Camp with classmates, neighbours, and their parents |
| 4 | Friends build Buddy System at home and community via after-school programs and playdates | Playdate with classmates – foster existing friendships and make new friends | Invite classmates and friends to the child's birthday party | Join other clubs that match with the child's hobby and interest to make new friends |
| 5 | Acquaintances and strangers met at home and in the community | Talk to a cashier during check-out in a supermarket | Participate verbally/non-verbally in a yard sale, lemonade stand, and flea market | Attend "Reading paws" with a talking buddy, and talk to strangers |

# Form 1.2 SMart Village – Name List of Helper

Anyone who is in the child's life

| | Group of people | Who can help | Buddy system (p25) | What can they do | Where can they help | When can they help |
|---|---|---|---|---|---|---|
| 1 | Parents and families | | | | | |
| 2 | Teachers and SM treating professional | | | | | |
| 3 | Classmates in buddy system | | | | | |
| 4 | Friends in buddy system | | | | | |
| 5 | Acquaintances and strangers | | | | | |

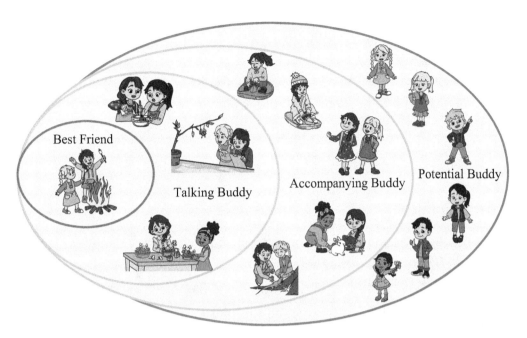

**FIGURE 1.4  Buddy system**

# Buddy System – Essential Component No. 6

Home is where children with SM can talk freely around people in their comfort zone. However, when they are in school or the community, they change into another person, isolated from the crowd. To help these children transition seamlessly from home to school to the community, consider building a rainbow bridge, a supporting system connecting the home to the outside world. The core of the rainbow bridge is a buddy system.

A buddy system serves as a "cocoon" that gently protects SM children from potential setbacks. It gives SM children a sense of security and supports them in the areas needed. Most importantly, a buddy system can help the voice of children with SM be heard outside of the home. The system is dynamic and can be personalised according to each child's condition and situation. A buddy system can be set up in different groups, as shown in the above cartoon and explained further in detail below. Nurture potential and accompanying buddies as they will become the talking buddies on the child's Rainbow Bridge.

1. **Potential buddy** whom the child wants to be friends with. Discuss with the child and ask the teacher about whom the child plays with in school and who is easy-going, and make a Name List of Classmates, Neighbours, and Friends.

2. **Accompanying buddy** whom the child does not yet talk to but can communicate with using gestures, e.g., accompanying to the bathroom, cafeteria, playground, gym, etc.
3. **Talking buddy** whom the child talks to. How loudly or quietly they talk depends on who else is around and how comfortable the child feels.
4. **Best friend** whom the child talks to and who always looks after and supports the child.

## Tips and Tricks

- The buddy system should be broad enough to cover every aspect of the child's life in which they encounter real issues.
- Expand potential buddy circle by making new friends. Foster each friendship to move more buddies from the outer circle into the inner circle. Form 1.3 helps parents to track the buddy system.
- Children might whisper to their talking buddies at first but should gradually get louder as they feel more comfortable. Accept whispering when it happens and respond as if the child has spoken at normal volume, but do not encourage whispering by telling children it's OK to whisper. This can lead to children relying on whispering, which can impede progress.

# Form 1.3 Buddy System Name List in/outside of School

|  | Name | Relationship (classmates/ neighbour/ friends) | Potential buddy | Accompanying buddy | Talking buddy | Best friends |
|---|---|---|---|---|---|---|
| 1 |  |  |  |  |  |  |
| 2 |  |  |  |  |  |  |
| 3 |  |  |  |  |  |  |
| 4 |  |  |  |  |  |  |
| 5 |  |  |  |  |  |  |
| 6 |  |  |  |  |  |  |
| 7 |  |  |  |  |  |  |
| 8 |  |  |  |  |  |  |
| 9 |  |  |  |  |  |  |
| 10 |  |  |  |  |  |  |

# Part 2

# PARENTS BECOME ADVOCATES INSIDE AND OUTSIDE OF SCHOOL

This section is for parents, who are the number one essential component in the recovery journey of children with selective mutism (SM). It provides various ways in which parents can support their child both in and outside of school.

When parents first learn of their child's SM, they often wonder where to start to help their child. In Parents Become Advocates, readers can find the suggestions and the steps to follow on the child's recovery journey. Table 2.1 summarises what parents can do, followed by a "Dos and Don'ts" list. In bringing pets to the school playground, readers can find the example of graded questions to engage the child in a conversation. The section raises awareness of the importance of spending quality time with the child, talking to the child about their SM, and making an action plan. Readers can also find a reward calendar and an example of taking small steps toward recovery.

To better facilitate the child's intervention, parents can consider volunteering in the school cafeteria, in-school gardening club, and after-school clubs such as Girl Scouts. Additionally, parents can prepare the child with a daily routine in advance to lower anxiety. Parents can use the slide-in/slide-out strategy to introduce new people through playful games with their child in the classroom corner. Playing games in the counsellor's office is also helpful if the school can provide the resource.

The authors hope that the practical examples in this section will inspire parents to step out of their comfort zone, be creative, and try new things to help and support their child both in and out of school. This includes participating in the school intervention plan setup, tracking the child's progress, monitoring their activity, and revising the action plan as the child's SM condition improves. The authors also encourage parents to be a positive influence in the lives of others while finding ways

DOI: 10.4324/9781003355267-2

to help their child. Building a community of people who understand SM and are willing to provide support in and out of school can benefit the child's recovery.

Not all of these ideas and suggestions will be possible to implement in your setting and some of them may not suit your child, but the section is designed to give you inspiration, and to show you what was effective for Amy.

The authors want to remind parents of the importance of advocacy, small steps, and a supportive environment in helping the child progress toward recovery.

# Parents Are the No. 1 Essential Component in SM Recovery Journey

## *Parents Become Advocates*

1. Parents study and educate others, including families, teachers, and friends, about SM. Parents openly discuss SM with the child using age-appropriate SM information. Parents also need to learn parenting skills to strengthen parent-child relationships.

2. Seek an SM treating professional who will provide a diagnosis and set up an intervention plan. If an SM treating professional is not accessible, parents need to take on the responsibility of the intervention.

3. Understand and support the child: find out the child's "Communication Stage" and various challenges. Identify the challenges that impact the child's health and safety. Give them the highest priority in terms of intervention. Practise and rehearse activities to help the child deal with daily tasks in school.

4. Parents and teachers set up a support plan and participate in the activities/events inside and outside of school: contact the school and discuss SM-related books, videos, and training to set up the support system in school. Organise events inside and outside of school, such as birthday parties, sports meet, New Year's party, talent show, day/overnight trip, camping, zoo-visit, etc. Parents spend time at school to help the child in the classroom, and at school events, before-school care, after-school care, and clubs. Parents and teachers know when and how to apply recommended strategies.

5. Where possible, parents volunteer in school (long-term, short-term, or seasonal): parents participate in programs hosted by the school or other organisations. Parents serve as a bridge to connect the child to others and provide talking opportunities for the child.

6. Parents/school could consider extra support to help the child inside and outside of school: improve language and social skills at home if the child faces the challenge of a second language or lacks social skills.

7. Build the buddy system via playdate and after-school program: parents request a list of classmates as well as the teacher's recommendation on which classmate is better matched for a playdate and friendship-building. (See more about playdate, games and activities, smart village, and buddy system in other sections of the book).

8. Help the child rehearse for conversations at school. Practise possible questions such as "What is your name?" "How old are you?" "Do you have a pet?" "Do you like to draw?" The child can practise his/her answers with a talking buddy, adults, and strangers. Avoid asking open-ended questions, and instead, ask the easier "Yes/No" and forced-choice questions, e.g., "X or Y?".

"After each wonderful step forward, we cannot sit back and wait for something else to happen. Waiting doesn't change anything. We need to build on each achievement and take action to move forwards – then we see change!"

Parents have a vital role in helping their children overcome SM. We rely on the kindness and understanding of our neighbours and the commitment and goodwill of school staff. It is not always easy to make time in school to repeat simple talking games or activities with staff and classmates, but this very effective strategy can save years of worry and planning and struggle down the line".[1]

## Note

1 Johnson, M. & Reitman, J. (2023). The selective mutism workbook for parents and professionals – small steps, big changes, Speechmark Publishing.

### Tips and Tricks

- The amount of information provided above may seem overwhelming for parents, as it contains a lot of details and implies that a considerable amount of time and effort is required. However, it is important for parents to remember to take things one step at a time and not set unrealistic goals.
- Progress can be made by taking small steps consistently, and it may be helpful to look back and see how far you've come.
- This information serves as a reminder that parents cannot rely solely on professionals and schools to handle everything. But instead, they need to take an active role and contribute to their child's progress.
- The support system in school can be EHCP (Education, Health and Care Plan)/ SEND (Special Education Needs) /IEP (Individualised Education Program) or equivalent. Even without EHCP/SEN/IEP, parents still need to request a support system in place.

**TABLE 2.1 Parents the No. 1 essential components in SM recovery journey**

| No. | What parents can do | Examples of parent support in and outside school | | |
|---|---|---|---|---|
| 1 | Educate yourself and others about SM. Work closely with SM treating professionals and school | Cooperate with an SM treating professional | Demonstrate SM strategies | Openly discuss SM with child. Plan tasks and goals with child |
| 2 | Understand the child's situation in school<br>• Communication stage<br>• Challenge-academic<br>• Challenge-health<br>• Strength-talents and skills | Use bathroom, have lunch, walk into school, submit homework | Strength: Talents and skills | Exam, music, gym, art, language |
| 3 | Parents and teachers set up a support plan | Play games in the classroom | Demonstrate voice exposure at home visit | Bake together at home visit |
| 4 | Parents volunteer in school (long-term, short-term, seasonal) | Volunteer in cafeteria | Volunteer in the school club programs | Volunteer in other non-profit organisations |
| 5 | Parent, shadow teacher, tutor, nanny, and coach support in after-school programs /clubs located both inside and outside of the school | Shadow teacher and classmates/ schoolmates | Tutor, teacher, and classmate | Coach, siblings, neighbours, and classmate |
| 6 | Build the buddy system through playdates and after-school programs | Meet classmates and other parents in school/ neighbourhood | Well-planned playdates and parties | Shopping with family/ friends |

## Parents' Dos and Don'ts List

**Do**

1. Accept the child for who he/she is. Understand that SM is an anxiety disorder, not a choice.
2. Educate yourself and others about SM and learn intervention strategies.
3. Communicate and team up with teachers, school officials, school counsellors, and/or psychologists for in-school intervention.
4. Do describe, praise, and if appropriate, reward your child's success.
5. Be patient. Allow 5 seconds for your child to prepare the answer and respond.
6. Learn and use strategies to facilitate your child's friendship-building and expand their circle of friends.
7. Have regular one-on-one or small group playdates at home and in your community. Playdates should be fun, exciting, long enough, and have parents involved. Start with one classmate and gradually increase the number of invitees. Parents may offer to help others, such as picking up/dropping off classmates.
8. Be aware of your own response to your child's silence. Check your facial expression and tone, do not make children think they are making you anxious, sad, or angry.
9. Discover your child's talent and make it shine.
10. Provide support and encourage your child to do things independently.
11. Understand and remember that small steps lead to big changes. Take small and gradual steps for SM intervention.
12. Always have a backup plan.
13. Volunteer to help in school and the community.
14. Stay positive and keep going even if progress seems slow or stalled.

1. Force, coax, or beg your child to talk.
2. Punish your child for not speaking.
3. Criticise your child.
4. Speak for your child.
5. Make a huge commotion when you first hear the child speaking.
6. Put the child in the spotlight.
7. Focus only on the child's silence and ignore other factors that impact their daily routine.
8. Set unrealistic goals that your child cannot achieve.
9. Give rewards for unmet goals.

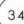

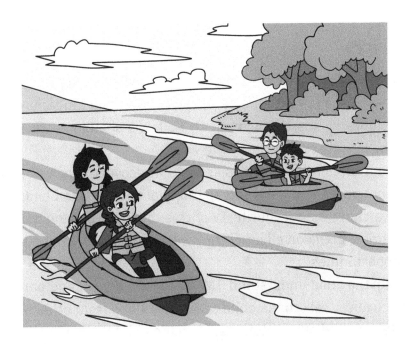

## Spending Quality Time with Your Child

Amy and her brother Tom planned a weekend kayaking trip for family time. Amy
was fully involved in purchasing, assembling, and pumping air into the kayak. She
was excited and took the credit for choosing a beautiful day for the trip. Amy and
Tom raced, joked, and shared what happened at school. Amy planned to invite
her friends to the next kayaking trip. Talking about friends, Amy began to tell Tom
whom she wanted to invite: girls in the Girl Scouts, friends from her dance club, and
classmates. When Amy grabbed a piece of water grass and pretended to throw it at
Tom, everyone dodged and laughed.

## Tips and Tricks

- After a stressful day in school, a child is often too exhausted to share anything that happened with the parent. A relaxed and fun family trip can help the child voluntarily share information. "Follow a snail for a walk, but do not forget the beautiful scenery along the way."

- A good parent-child relationship is key to SM recovery. It is never too late to learn about parenting skills and spend quality time with children. For example, watching their favourite TV shows together, playing games, reading bedtime stories, going on a family trip, and even grocery shopping offer bonding opportunities.

- Parents help the child understand SM, build confidence, and participate in different activities. Talk to the child about reactions from others. Discuss daily challenges and offer solutions. Help the child build a buddy system both inside and outside of school.

- Motivate the child by setting up an incentive system where the child can enjoy their favourite activities after achieving goals.

- Rehearsing activities/situations/conversations in advance can help the child gain a firm foundation for courage, confidence, and self-esteem.

- Share the experiences at school via video recording (see more on pages 112 & 193)

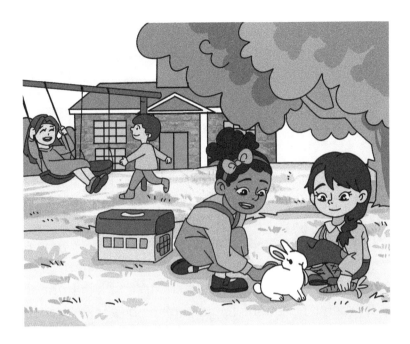

## Bringing Pets to the School Playground

Although school had just started, most of Amy's classmates had given up talking to her because she never responded to their questions. In order to provide Amy an opportunity to interact verbally with her classmates, Amy's mom brought Amy's pet bunny "Fluffy" to the school playground one day after school. Amy played with and fed Fluffy carrots. To reduce anxiety, Amy and her mom agreed on an escape route. If too many classmates asked questions, Amy could leave and go to the swing.

Once they saw the bunny, Amy's classmates began to gather around, but they only talked to Amy's mom. Amy's mom told them the bunny was Amy's, and they could ask Amy questions.

At first, Amy responded by nodding and shaking her head when asked, "Is this your bunny?" and "Can I pet your bunny?" To help Amy answer verbally, Amy's mom repeated the questions and waited for a few seconds for Amy to respond to her rather than the children. Sometimes, mom said the first part of the sentence and let Amy complete the rest, e.g., "Fluffy likes to run, jump, and... " Amy would then say, "sleep." Other times, mom rephrased the questions as forced-choice questions, e.g., "Does Fluffy like carrot or cabbage?" Slowly, Amy could also answer simple questions like "Where does Fluffy sleep?" Amy's mom stepped away and let Amy interact with her classmates on her own. Soon enough, Amy joined her classmates in playing and chasing on the playground.

For the remaining year, Amy took guinea pigs, birds, turtles, and chicks to the school playground! Her circle of friends expanded. These friends became her talking buddies in school, at home, and in the community.

## Tips and Tricks

- The school playground is a great place to meet other parents and arrange playdates. Amy's mom can use this opportunity to talk openly about Amy's SM, educate others about SM, and ask genuinely for help from other parents.
- In addition to playdates at home or in the community, Amy can join after-school clubs and other activities that her classmates attend.
- Use this graded question sequence to help children talk in front of other people gradually: Yes/no questions (child can nod or shake head in response); choice questions (child answers with a single word); closed questions (e.g., Who? What? Where?) requiring single words, then phrases; open-ended questions (e.g., Why? How?). When the child responds successfully and comfortably, move on to the next type of question (also see page 76). If there is no response after five seconds, rephrase the question at the previous level or move on with a friendly comment.

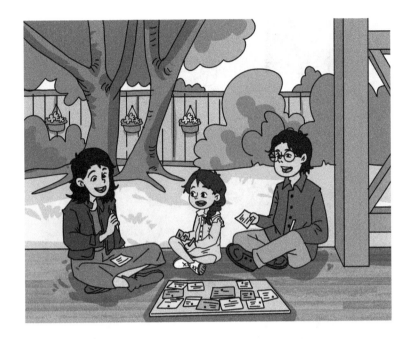

## Child's Participation – the Essential Component No. 8 – Talk to Amy about Her SM and Make an Action Plan

"Why don't you talk?" "You talk to me outside of school. Why don't you talk to me in school?" Amy heard these kinds of questions all the time. It was important that we talked openly to Amy about her SM and tried to find out what aspects of her day created anxiety for her. "You have been trying really hard to talk to your friend Sofie for a long time. How did it feel when you couldn't get your words out today?...You did nothing wrong. Let me tell you a secret: I used to not talk in school, just like you. You will talk if you let it come gradually. It is just a matter of time."

We then went through Amy's day with her to find out what was easy and what could be difficult and tried to come up with a solution together. For example, Amy missed her stop when a substitute driver was on duty. Mom sat her next to James on the school bus, so Amy had someone help her relay the message in case she needed to speak to the driver. With the teacher's help, Amy was paired with a buddy to accompany her for issues with daily routine: going to the bathroom with Isabella, eating lunch with Cate.

We explained to Amy that things would get easier for her if she did small things, a little bit at a time, such as, helping out in the technology class, going to Gardening club after school on Monday, submitting the Ski club application form, sending out birthday invitations, only talking to one new person at a time. She could repeatedly practise the same tasks with the same classmates/friends, and then add new people to expand the talking circle.

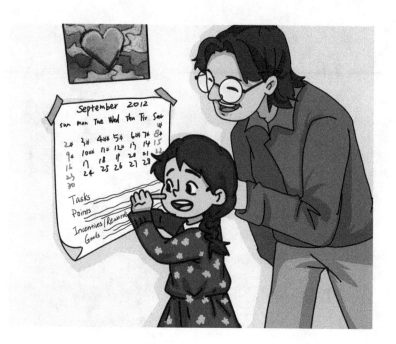

## Reward Calendar
### Complete Tasks, Earn Points, Redeem Rewards and Achieve Goals

"Daddy, I did it! I walked into school by myself this morning!" Amy shared the good news with her dad once she got home. "Well done, Amy, you walked into school by yourself! (positive reinforcement with labelled praise). Walking into school has been difficult for you. But you did it today! You can put a star on the calendar now." Amy's dad said encouragingly. Every month, Amy and her parents would make a plan to list tasks, points, rewards, and goals that she agreed to on the calendar. Amy was more motivated to work hard and felt supported rather than pressured. Once Amy reached a certain number of points, she could choose a reward. It could be being the boss for a day, feeding ducks in the pond, a pajama playdate, making cookies for the class party and so on.

At night, Amy eagerly reported on the day's tasks, put a sticker or drew a star on her calendar, and then calculated the points. This calendar served as a visual record of Amy's progress and helped her parents track how she was doing. Amy's progress was based not on whether or not she spoke, but on the things she had never dared to do before. She earned points every day, and her parents would praise her by describing specifically the task that Amy accomplished.

## Tips and Tricks

- Goals should be specific and meaningful to the child.
- Avoid bribing – goals will only be achieved if they are realistic – bribes won't help.
- Tasks should be set up based on the child's challenge and daily work.
- Keep goals simple – the child may lose motivation if it takes too long or is too difficult to earn the reward.
- Be consistent in giving out rewards.
- Rewards don't have to be large or expensive! Choosing a favourite film or helping to select and cook a family meal could be options. The key is to motivate rather than bribe.
- Success ultimately becomes its own reward.

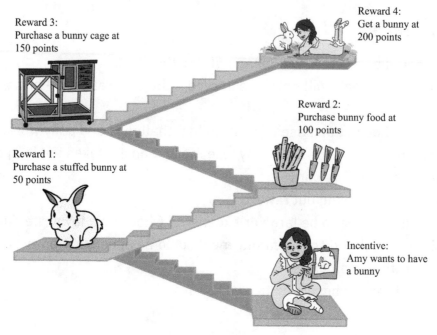

**FIGURE 2.1** Set up tasks, earn points, redeem rewards and achieve goals

## Rewards, Goals, and Incentives

Not all children respond well to task-setting and rewards. They first need to experience success and be proud of their achievements to enjoy this approach, so be guided by your child.

The non-verbal tasks include waving, receiving, passing, collecting, going to the bathroom, eating in school, doing schoolwork, handing in homework, and using gestures. The verbal tasks include using sounds, talking to adults via the talking buddies, reading, and answering questions. Breaking down the task into smaller pieces of success was difficult to achieve.

Long-term goals may be accumulated from short-term goals. For example, the long-term goal is to initiate conversation and freely talk to classmates; the short-term goal is to make more friends and answer their questions. Pair practice with positive reinforcement, including specific praise ("Thank you for letting me know...) and tangible reinforcers (stickers, check marks, and prizes). Build in enjoyable activities to celebrate their achievements, but avoid a deadline as the added time pressure is counter-productive. Sometimes a light remark is helpful, e.g., "I'll have to be careful – when you can talk to the server yourself, you'll be able to order ice cream AND a milkshake!" It is also helpful if parents reinforce their child's bravery when they come home, so be sure to have a communication method, such as a communication book, to relay information about progress and any setbacks.

Figure 2.1 provides an illustrative example of establishing a reward and incentive system through goal-setting. It is important for parents and the child to discuss goals, rewards, tasks, and associated points values to prioritise challenges. For example, tasks like talking to a classmate could be worth five points, while simply waving a greeting to teachers could be worth one point.

Track the progress and count the points daily. When the child accumulates a certain number of points, they can choose to redeem rewards. The child will be more motivated to work hard towards their goals, exhibiting brave behaviours. Form 2.1a shows an example of weekly tasks and points recording. Use it together with the communication task book (Form 3.1) to record the child's weekly progress. Parents can note the child's communication stage, achievement, challenges, and setbacks at the end of the week, which helps with task planning.

## Form 2.1a Communication Steps Tasks, Points, Rewards, and Goals Weekly

### Goal: Navigate the School Life

|   | TASK | Points | M | TU | W | TH | F | Sat | Sun |
|---|------|--------|---|----|----|----|----|-----|-----|
| 1 | Go to the toilet/bathroom | 5 | | | | | | | |
| 2 | Eat and drink in school | 5 | | | | | | | |
| 3 | Walk in school without help | 8 | | | | | | | |
| 4 | Submit homework | 9 | | | | | | | |
| 5 | Participate in activity | 10 | | | | | | | |

# Form 2.1 Communication Steps Tasks, Points, Rewards, and Goals Weekly

**Goal:**

| | TASK | Points | M | TU | W | TH | F | Sat | Sun |
|---|---|---|---|---|---|---|---|---|---|
| 1 | | | | | | | | | |
| 2 | | | | | | | | | |
| 3 | | | | | | | | | |
| 4 | | | | | | | | | |
| 5 | | | | | | | | | |
| 6 | | | | | | | | | |
| 7 | | | | | | | | | |
| Total Point – Daily | | | | | | | | | |
| Total Point – Weekly | | | | | | | | | |

## Reward for

1. 20 points for
2. 40 points for
3. 60 points for
4. 80 points for
5. 100 points for

**Note:**

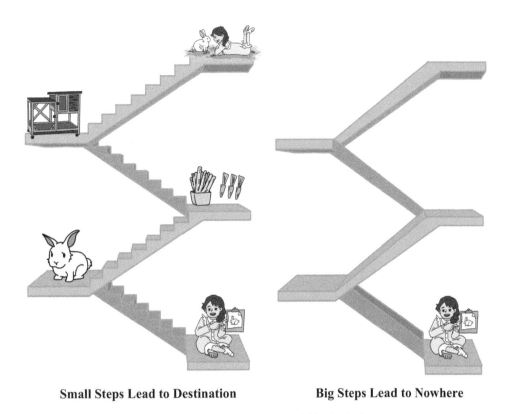

**Small Steps Lead to Destination**   **Big Steps Lead to Nowhere**

**FIGURE 2.2** Small steps lead to destination and big steps lead to? (Setbacks)

Go one little step at a time, don't set your goals too high.

In the left picture, Amy really wanted a bunny. In order for her to get that bunny, Amy agreed with her parents that she had to achieve different goals. Each goal was further broken down into small tasks that Amy was more capable of doing. She earned points after completing each task. As she reached certain points, Amy could trade in for a small reward or accumulate the points for a bigger prize. Some of these tasks were easy, and others were not. But by completing these tasks, Amy became braver and more confident. In the end, Amy completed all of her goals and received the ultimate reward, her dream bunny.

In the right picture, Amy also wanted a bunny. But this BIG goal could not be accomplished since there were no **SMALL STEPS** in place to support her getting there.

A common question that parents ask is, "How come I did everything that I could, but nothing seemed to change?" Parents need to consider whether the assigned task or goal is realistic.

## Tips and Tricks

- Small steps: the tasks are based on the child's capability and are SMALL enough that the child can work on them to achieve different goals.
- Big steps: the assigned tasks are too complex for the child to accomplish, which may discourage the child from trying new tasks and may lead to regression.

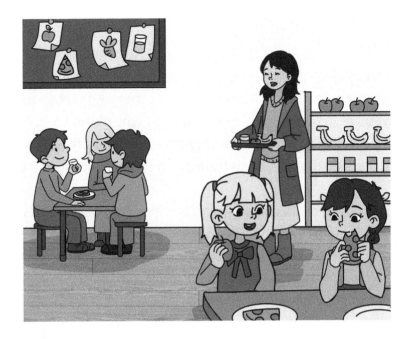

## Parents Volunteer at School – Cafeteria

Amy and Mom agreed to use lunchtime to make more friends. Amy's mom was a member of the Parent Teacher Association (PTA) and volunteered at the school's cafeteria. Mom assured Amy that she would join Amy at lunchtime to support her.

The next day in the cafeteria, Amy, her talking buddy Sofie, and Amy's mom chose a corner table to eat their lunch. They played the Wiz Kidz game afterward. Feeling curious, a few of Amy's classmates came over to check out the game. "What are you playing?" one classmate asked. "It's a game called Wiz Kidz," answered Sofie. Amy nodded in agreement. "Where did you get this game?" another classmate asked. "Amy got it from her grandparents for Christmas. Right, Amy?" Mom made a mistake intentionally. "No...birthday," Amy said in a whisper.

From that day on, they played other interesting and fun games at lunchtime, which attracted different classmates to join them. Sometimes, Amy and her mom would show videos of Amy's playdates with her talking buddies baking cookies at home, feeding birds in the park, and camping in the mountains. Seeing how active and talkative Amy was outside of school, Amy's classmates all wanted to have playdates with her. Slowly but steadily, Amy made more friends and talked to each of them at lunchtime. Once Amy spoke confidently, Mom left the dining table to help in the kitchen.

## Tips and Tricks

- Talking in the classroom in front of their peers can be overwhelming for SM children. Parents, teachers, keyworkers, or other supportive adults can help the child speak in other parts of school first where the child feels less scrutinised, e.g., school's playground, cafeteria, counsellor's office, etc. Once the child speaks, the adult can then bring the conversations into the classroom.
- Parents or supportive adults can serve as a bridge that connects SM children to a new person. Support the child to answer questions by waiting 5 seconds before repeating and/or rephrasing questions.

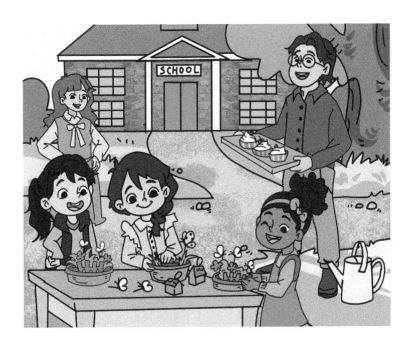

## Parents Volunteer at School – Gardening Club

When Amy joined the after-school gardening club hosted by her teacher Ms. Alice, Amy's dad volunteered to carry soil, deliver water, and clean the site. Dad asked Amy to help him deliver water to her friends and told her, "You can ask your friends whether they need water by saying, 'need water?' or 'water?' They all know you can talk at home." When Amy shook her head, Dad said, "Don't worry, you can just talk to me until it feels easier. You can tell me your friends' names, then I'll see who needs more water, and you can hand them the watering can."

Dad sometimes would bring treats, such as cupcakes, to the club. He even took the children to the local ice cream shop after the club once. The children were super excited and eager to get their favourite toppings for their ice cream. Amy ordered her ice cream using her talking bird, a recording device that pre-recorded her order message at home. Amy and her friends played with the talking bird by recording and playing funny messages. Everyone was having a good time. On the ride home, Amy responded to her friends behind her talking bird. No recording was needed!

## Tips and Tricks

- Parents can use their knowledge, work experiences, talents, and interests to be more involved in school and after-school programs. For example, parents can help at a school club like computer coding, music, gardening, woodwork. Often any help is valued, even if you don't consider it an area of expertise!

- Parents can help the child explore opportunities for volunteer work (individual or group), which is beneficial not only for social and conversational skills but also for self-esteem enhancement.

- Parents assure the child that it is safe to talk in public. If the child is unable to talk, parents can step away from the crowd to where the child can speak freely. This is better than allowing children to whisper in their parent's ear as if talking is 'banned'. In time, the distance between the child and the crowd decreases.

- Once children are able to talk to their parents in front of their friends, it is much easier for them to start talking to their friends, too.

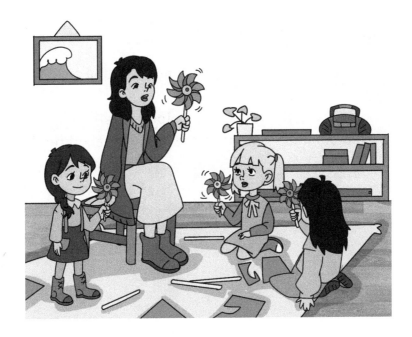

## Parents Volunteer at After-school Club – Girl Scouts

To further help Amy get involved in group activities, Amy's mom became a troop leader at Girl Scout Troop 80602. Girl Scout members, a group of Amy's classmates and schoolmates, would meet twice a month after school, either in school or offsite. They were involved in all kinds of fun and meaningful activities, e.g., picking pumpkins, cleaning the local stream, harvesting corn, and spending the night at the aquarium. Amy made many friends from Girl Scouts over the years. They became her talking buddies and best friends both inside and outside of school.

At one of the Girl Scouts events, Amy's mom led the girls to make wind wheels to be donated at the local community event. Amy helped Mom distribute paper, sticks, glue, and scissors. "Oh no, my paper is ripped!" Rosa called out. "Amy, can you please go and check on Rosa to see what she needs?" Mom asked. "Can you please ask Leah to put the extra materials in the box?" Mom tried to provide talking opportunities for Amy to talk to children individually before speaking in front of the whole group. Sometimes, Mom intentionally made mistakes, and Amy would speak up to correct her. In the beginning, Amy would respond to her mom and answer friends' questions in a few words. As she got more comfortable, she was able to talk spontaneously in front of her friends. When they were done, the girls blew on the wind wheels to see whose spun the fastest.

## Tips and Tricks

- Parents or supportive adults provide opportunities for the child to actively participate in group activities.
- After the child joins the activity, they are helped to talk to familiar adults and friends in front of others until they are ready to talk directly to other people.

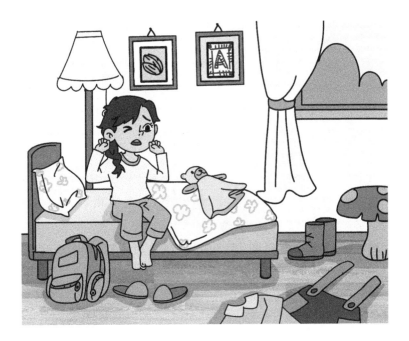

## Preparing for Going to School in the Morning

Amy had trouble falling asleep at night and waking up in the morning. Even if she got up on time, she was slow to get ready for school. Amy's mom found that the anxiety about going to school was the real cause behind all these problems.

To help Amy lower her anxiety, her mom made a few adjustments. First, the night before, Mom helped Amy familiarise herself with the daily routine by looking together at the school schedule, after-school program, and any possible schedule changes. Then, Mom built a buddy system for Amy and told her, "Amy, your bus and bathroom buddy Isabella, lunch buddy Cate, and break time/recess buddy Marisa are all in school today." Lastly, Mom reassured Amy that nobody would make her talk in school and all her worries had been taken care of. For example, Mom told Amy, "Teachers will only ask you questions in class if you put your hand up."; "You don't have to sing, you can play an instrument instead."; "Your clothes are all set."; "Your homework is in your school bag."; "When you line up for the bus, stand in front of your talking buddy Cate."; "Mom will pick you up at the bus stop, and we will go to the ballet class together afterward."

## Tips and Tricks

- SM takes time to overcome, but urgent issues need to be addressed immediately, such as using the bathroom, eating lunch, reporting injuries, submitting homework, etc. The buddy system can usually fix these issues quickly, e.g., an accompanying buddy can walk the child with SM to the bathroom on a set schedule.
- Use various forms of communication. Prepare a photo album with pictures of the toilet, cafeteria, stomach pain, parent's phone number, etc. Children with SM can point to the pictures to convey their needs.
- Record greetings and daily conversations on a "voice-recording toy" at home and play the recordings when needed.
- The child talks through toys, puppets, or animals. Bring a puppet or a stuffed animal that SM children can hide behind and talk using their own voice. Adults direct their questions to the toy instead, such as "Do you know what Amy would like to drink?"

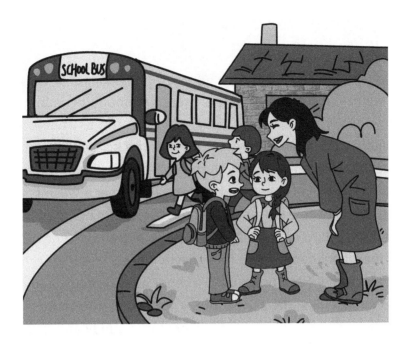

## Riding the School Bus and Bus Buddy

Riding the school bus had never been easy for Amy. Things got worse on the day a substitute bus driver took over unexpectedly. Not knowing Amy's condition and her home stop, the substitute bus driver did not wait for Amy to get off before driving on. Amy missed her bus stop and was too scared to say anything until her classmate Isabella offered to take Amy to her home. Amy's mom panicked when her daughter did not arrive home on time and started calling Amy's classmates. Luckily, Mom was able to locate Amy after dialling Isabella's number. Mom decided to find a bus buddy for Amy to prevent incidents like this from happening again. The next day, at the school bus stop, Amy's mom asked her neighbour and classmate, James, "Can you remind Amy to get off the bus with you on the way home?" James said, "Of course!" In addition, Amy brought her monkey, a talking toy with a voice message pre-recorded at home. Amy could squeeze the monkey's hand to play the recording when needed, "I get off at Clinton stop. Please call my mom if I missed my stop."

## Tips and Tricks

- A buddy system should be diverse and cover every aspect of SM children's life that they have real issues in. In Amy's case, a school bus buddy helps to solve her problems easily.

- Help SM children familiarise themselves with the school bus route. Rehearse and practise daily conversations with the school bus driver at home, such as "hello" and "thank you," and let children know that a wave is fine until their voice pops out easily. Prepare a name tag and contact info card with SM children's name, photo, home address, and guardian's phone number. Put the card in their backpack where it is easy to access in an emergency.

- Educate others about SM. Contact the school bus company and inform them about an SM child riding the school bus. Offer them information on dos and don'ts, e.g., let the child sit with their school bus buddy and feel free to smile and say hello, but don't expect the child to respond verbally.

## Sliding-in

Use the sliding-in strategy to make it easier for the child to accept a new person into their talking circle. The child's progress depends on several factors. Some children will open up more quickly, and some may need the process broken down into smaller steps. Sliding-in may need to be repeated several times with the same adult/classmate until the child can talk to them. When introducing a new person, begin with someone who will help the child facilitate future sliding-ins, such as a keyworker. It may take a few tries/months to complete these steps and see results. Move to the next step only when the current step succeeds. To accelerate the progress, observe the situation, keep the momentum when moving up, and be patient when moving down.

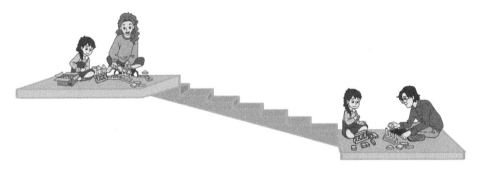

**FIGURE 2.3 Sliding-in**

| | |
|---|---|
| 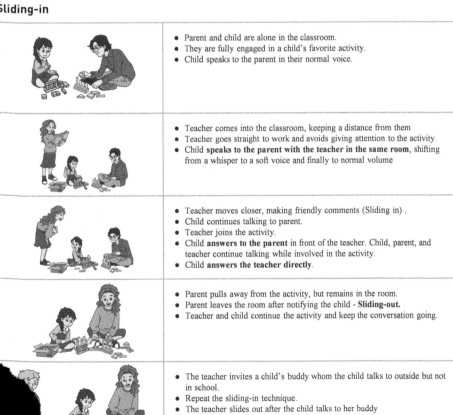 | • Parent and child are alone in the classroom.<br>• They are fully engaged in a child's favorite activity.<br>• Child speaks to the parent in their normal voice. |
| | • Teacher comes into the classroom, keeping a distance from them<br>• Teacher goes straight to work and avoids giving attention to the activity.<br>• Child **speaks to the parent with the teacher in the same room**, shifting from a whisper to a soft voice and finally to normal volume |
| | • Teacher moves closer, making friendly comments (Sliding in) .<br>• Child continues talking to parent.<br>• Teacher joins the activity.<br>• Child **answers to the parent** in front of the teacher. Child, parent, and teacher continue talking while involved in the activity.<br>• Child **answers the teacher directly**. |
| | • Parent pulls away from the activity, but remains in the room.<br>• Parent leaves the room after notifying the child - **Sliding-out.**<br>• Teacher and child continue the activity and keep the conversation going. |
| | • The teacher invites a child's buddy whom the child talks to outside but not in school.<br>• Repeat the sliding-in technique.<br>• The teacher slides out after the child talks to her buddy |

...mal version of The Sliding-in Technique, developed by Maggie Johnson (1997).[2]

Note: This is an infor...

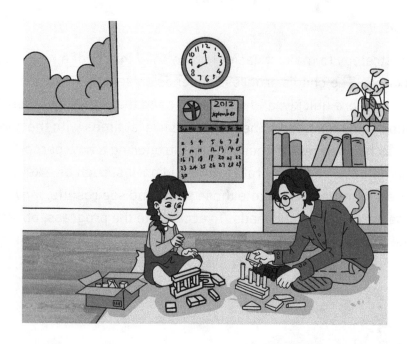

## Dad Playing Games with Amy in the Classroom Corner

Dad and Amy had tried to arrive at school before everyone else in the morning.

It would give them a little time to play games and read books together in the empty classroom. One evening when Dad told Amy that they would play in the classroom tomorrow, Amy jumped up with joy. But then she became concerned. "What if others want to join us and play too?" "You can decide whether to let them play with us," Dad reassured Amy.

The next morning, they brought Amy's favourite wooden building blocks to school. They set the blocks in the classroom corner, far away from the door, to avoid being disturbed when others came in. "Amy, do you want to build a bridge?" Dad asked. "Ok, how about building a tall bridge, just like the one we passed yesterday?" Amy replied while playing with her building blocks.

## Note

2  Johnson, M. & Wintgens, A. (1997). The selective mutism resource manual, Speechmark Practical.

## Trick and Tips

- Parents act as a talking bridge to bring the child's voice to school.
- Parents help the child practise at home and become good at the activity that they can later bring to school or a playdate.
- Recommend parent-child interactions in school in line with what the school will allow. It would be best if inviting classmates and teachers to the activity.
- Before class starts in the morning: the parent and child spend time together in the empty classroom until the teacher and students walk in.
- During recess or lunch break: e.g., parent volunteers at the school canteen and helps the child eat and interact in a relaxed setting.
- After school: parents can come into the classroom to read with the child when no one is around. Or they can play in the school's playground.

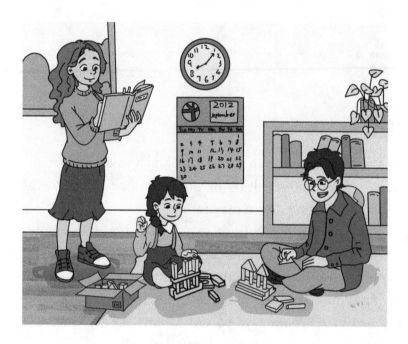

## Introduce a New Person into the Game

Amy really enjoyed playing with her dad in the classroom before everyone came in the morning. She talked comfortably with Dad when no one was around. It was time to introduce Ms. Carole to their morning game. When Ms. Carole entered the classroom, she went to get busy with her work. She did not pay attention or talk to Amy. Dad and Amy continued playing. "How many layers are you building?" Dad asked. Amy remained silent, afraid to be heard by Ms. Carole. After a short pause, Dad rephrased the question, "Are you going to stick with two layers?" Amy nodded.

After seeing Ms. Carole busy with her tasks and keeping a distance from them, Amy lowered her guard. Dad tried a choice question, "Do you like yours or mine best?" "Mine, of course!" Amy answered in a soft voice but with a grin. "Why is that?" Dad added to create more talking opportunities. "Because mine is bigger, taller, stronger, and better looking!" Amy made a funny face at her dad.

Ms. Carole started to walk towards them. "Wow, it looks like you are building a beautiful palace, Amy. I love how you're doing that. And Dad's looks like my house," Ms. Carole commented. Amy looked up at Ms. Carole and smiled. "I wonder who's going to finish first?" Ms. Carole continued making comments without expecting responses or eye contact from Amy. (This is known as commentary style talking/ sportscaster).

## Tips and Tricks

- When a new person is introduced to an activity, they should keep a distance from the child in the beginning and pretend to be busy. The new person can gradually approach the child after the child is comfortable enough to talk in their presence.
- Only one new person, either a teacher or classmate, is introduced each time. This will prevent the child from getting overwhelmed or anxious.
- The new person should make friendly comments initially rather than asking questions and expecting the child to talk. This is called "commentary-style talk/Sportscaster." It includes chatty, rhetorical questions that need no answer.
- Parents use graded questions to ease children into talking in front of other people (see pages 38 & 76).

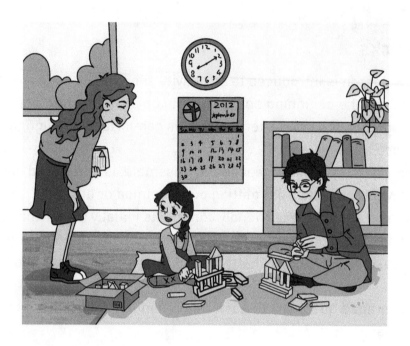

## New Person Slides In

Ms. Carole waited until Amy talked to Dad again and then tried another question. "Does your building have a name?" Ms. Carole asked. Amy stared at Dad and shrugged her shoulders. "Is it a palace or a tower?" Dad asked. "Tower," Amy whispered to Dad and then corrected herself, "No, castle!" "Wow, that's even better than a palace," Ms. Carole said. "Have you ever visited a castle?" Amy nodded, looking directly at Ms. Carole. Ms. Carole got down on the floor with Dad and Amy. "I'd love to go to a real castle," Ms. Carole continued. "Is this going to be a two-layer or three-layer castle?" "Two," Amy replied in a whisper.

"OK, well, it looks like your dad's nearly finished. But if we team up, I think we can finish your castle faster than his. I'd love to help." Amy smiled at her teacher. "What shape do we need next?" Ms. Carole asked. "A triangle," Amy answered in a more audible voice. Ms. Carole rummaged in the box and passed a triangle to Amy.

## Tips and Tricks

- Allow the child to talk comfortably to their parent or talking buddy before asking direct questions.
- A competitive game emphasising fun rather than talking often gets the child more excited and willing to participate.
- To build rapport, show genuine interest in the activity, and team up with the child for a common goal.
- Passing over and taking over items, such as building bricks in the above example, can help the child build rapport and non-verbal interaction with a new person.
- 5-second rule: When someone asks the child a question, parents should wait 5 seconds and resist the temptation to answer for the child. If there is no response, the parent then quietly rephrases the question as a yes/no or choice question and waits for another 5 seconds, allowing the child to respond to their parent with a nod or shake of the head or a single word. The parent repeats their answer if necessary. As children improve, the parent simply repeats the question, and the child answers them with one or more words. Soon, children will start to answer within the first 5-second period.

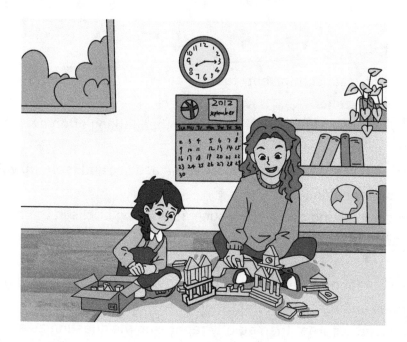

## Parent Slides Out

After seeing Amy and Ms. Carole playing and talking comfortably together, Dad quietly left the game. He went to organise the bookshelf and then picked a book to read nearby. Amy and Ms. Carole moved on to build a bridge. "Do you want to build a long or short bridge?" Ms. Carole asked. Amy shrugged.

"You are not sure? Ok then, let's build a long one with the arch." "This one?" asked Amy, reaching into the box. "How about the straight arch?" replied Ms.Carole, "I think it's longer." Amy looked again. "This is like the bridge I saw with Dad," she said, suddenly talking more easily.

Classmates began to walk in and came over to check out Amy and Ms. Carole's bridge. "Amy, it's time for me to go to work. I'll come back with your favourite game when school finishes at 3 pm." Amy's dad waved goodbye to her and left.

Ms. Carole asked Amy to invite one of her talking buddies to join the game. Once they began to talk, Ms. Carole asked Amy to invite one of her accompanying buddies to join them and left them to it. "I'll be over there if you need me." Ms. Carole assured Amy.

## Tips and Tricks

- The parent/talking buddy/teacher should serve as a talking bridge between the new person and the child. Slide out only after the child can comfortably talk to the new person.
- Parents should find an excuse to slide out as soon as possible, so children do not rely on them to facilitate conversation. Let the child know before leaving completely and assure them you will be back.

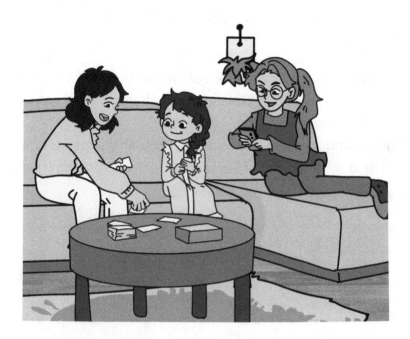

## Playing Games in Counsellor's Office

The new school year had started for a while, and Amy had settled into her new school. To help Amy accelerate her recovery progress, the school's counsellor, Ms. Christina, invited Amy and her mom to her office. Amy and her mom were playing Amy's favourite card game, UNO. Ms. Christina was watching Amy's Girl Scout Camporee video next to them. Ms. Christina giggled and commented on the video, "Amy and Marisa's boat is so much faster than Mom's boat." "Yes, the girls won the boat race." said Mom. Ms. Christina continued to watch the video without looking at or talking to Amy directly. "Yellow 3." Mom put down her card. "Yellow 8," Amy whispered. "Switch to red." Mom put down a red 8 card. "Uh-oh, I can't go." Amy muttered and drew a card from the pile. After a few rounds, Amy's voice became louder and louder.

And finally, she called out, "UNO!" using her excited voice.

## Tips and Tricks

- Identify a keyworker/supporter in school. Use the parent as a talking bridge: the child first talks to the parent in the keyworker/ supporter's presence and gradually talks directly to them.
- Meet with the keyworker/supporter one-on-one in a private space. Play a video of the child to get voice exposure: The child gets used to their voice being heard with no pressure to speak to the new person.
- Engage the child in an interesting and fun activity that will lead to verbal communication.

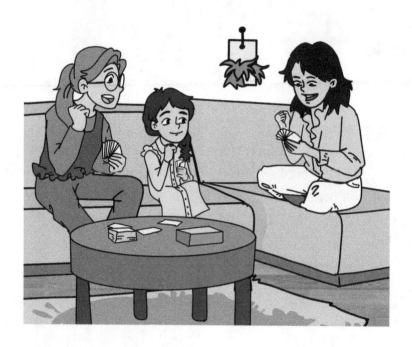

## Counsellor and Amy Teamed Up

After seeing Amy comfortably playing and talking with mom, Ms. Christina commented, "This is a cool game. I've never played it before. Is it difficult to learn?" "Amy, do you think it's a hard game?" Mom directed the question to Amy. Amy shook her head. "Can you teach me how to play, Amy? Maybe we can team up against your mom." Ms. Christina said to Amy with a wink. Amy nodded. Ms. Christina then switched her seat with Mand sat next to Amy. "Okay, let's see if I can work this out. If Mom played this card, could this card go down next?" asked Ms. Christina. Amy burst out laughing and shook her head. "How about this one?" "No," said Amy, looking at Mom, "only a two or a red one." Even though Ms. Christina was screaming in her head that Amy had answered, she tried to hold back her excitement and act calmly. "Ah, you match the colour or the number. Thank you!" Amy carried on explaining to Ms. Christina how to play and was soon making direct eye contact. "UNO!" Amy and Ms. Christina called out in unison. "Can we play Go Fish now, Mom?" asked Amy, not wanting the session to end. After a round of Go Fish, Mom made an excuse to go to the restroom and promised to come back soon, leaving Amy and Ms. Christina to play against each other.

## Tips and Tricks

- Team up with the child using humour whenever possible to quickly build rapport.
- Keyworker/supporter slides in/joins the game gradually, giving the child time to fully warm up, and is careful to use more comments than questions.
- Parent acts as a talking bridge to facilitate conversation.
- Practice turn-taking games at home that require talking, e.g., players describe or request cards, ask questions, or give clues. Other people can then join in.
- Parent slides out when the child can talk to the keyworker/supporter so that the child doesn't become reliant on their presence.

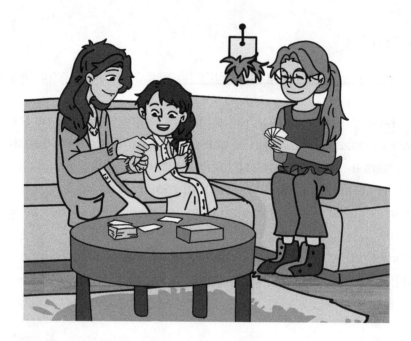

## Counsellor Practised SM Strategies

Ms. Christina wanted to continue the momentum of Amy's talking. She invited the maths teacher Ms. Pear to her office. Ms. Christina and Amy were playing cards while Ms. Pear sat aside and watched a video of Ms. Christina and Amy playing cards together. Amy had learned that it helped to make talking easier if other people heard her voice first. Later, Ms. Pear joined them. "Amy, who won the last game, Ms. Christina or you?" asked Ms. Pear. Amy looked at Ms. Christina and hesitated. Ms. Christina smiled and waited a few seconds. "Was it me or you?" she said. "Me," said Amy quietly, holding her gaze. "Yes, Amy's very good at this. I'm going to have to practise more," joked Ms. Christina. "Can you teach me how to play too? Then maybe I can practise with Ms. Christina." Ms. Pear suggested. With previous experience teaching Ms. Christina, Amy nodded confidently. After a few rounds, Amy could comfortably talk to Ms. Pear and even shared a joke with her.

## Tips and Tricks

- When people see how effective the result is after applying the right strategies, they are more willing to self-educate and educate others about SM knowledge.
- The child needs small steps to build confidence and gradually enable them to talk in front of different people and in various situations. For example, use structured activities and games with simple, rehearsed language rather than general conversation to help the child open up and release their voice. Practise at home first. Allow the child to speak comfortably to their talking partner before asking them questions. Ask graded questions (see pages 38 & 76); Change one thing at a time (e.g., repeat the same game but with a NEW person).
- Keep the momentum of talking going. Once the child starts to talk, keyworker/supporter invites different teachers and classmates to the office so that the child can talk to them in a private space. Gradually move the activities from the office to other areas of the school, such as the playground, cafeteria, classroom, etc.

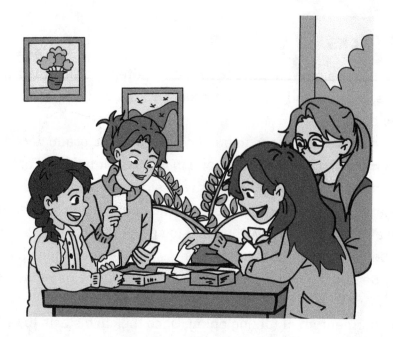

## Amy's Talking Circle Gets Expanded

Ms. Christina slid out when Ms. Pear and Amy could talk freely. Ms. Pear chatted with Amy about classwork, playdates, birthday party, movie night, and field trip. Amy's true colours shone through during these interactive sessions. "Amy, do you like turtles? Let's go check out the turtles in the pond next to the school garden." Ms. Pear said to Amy. "Can I invite my friend Marissa?" Amy replied. "Sure! But who is Marissa? Is she your friend? Does she go to Girl Scouts with you?" Ms. Pear asked question after question now that Amy was in talking mode.

Ms. Christina now wanted to help Amy get used to talking in larger groups. She invited Ms. Lisanne, the language teacher, to join them. Amy and Ms. Lisanne teamed up to compete against Ms. Christina and Ms. Pear to play 2v2 UNO. Amy explained to Ms. Lisanne about the game and its rules. She even told Ms. Lisanne about the plan to visit turtles!

## Tips and Tricks

- Spend one-on-one time with teachers and classmates in a private space to build rapport. Keep the conversation going by starting in a private room, continuing in the hallway, and finishing in the classroom.
- When the child starts to speak to her teacher one-on-one, the teacher may think she is over SM since the child can speak now. They don't realise that this is just the beginning of overcoming SM. There is still a long way to go until the child can speak spontaneously in any situation.
- Remember all of these techniques take time and practice, changes won't happen overnight but small steps will help.

# Part 3

# SCHOOL STAFF PROVIDING SUPPORT INSIDE AND OUTSIDE OF SCHOOL

This section highlights the vital role of teachers, the third essential component, in the recovery journey of children with selective mutism (SM). It offers practical guidance on how teachers can support these students both in and outside of school.

It includes tables summarising the strategies to use, the challenges children with SM face, and the support teachers and staff can provide in their recovery journey. A sample letter that can be sent to school gives parents a guide to write their own personal letters. Additionally, a "Dos and Don'ts" list for teachers is available for printing and giving to the teacher.

The emphasis is on the importance of easing students' transitions by visiting the new school before the new school year/term/semester, attending back-to-school evenings, and participating in moving up days before the school year ends. Other strategies for building rapport between teachers and students include private time with a counsellor or buddy, teacher's home visits, and teachers participating in the child's activities, as and when possible.

Although some supports, such as a shadow teacher, may not be provided by the school or any special education service, it is a powerful method for helping the child build rapport with teachers and classmates and for the teacher to employ various strategies, such as voice exposure, slide-in, and talking bridge. Parents may ask the school to give them a week or month to try it out and show that dramatic improvement can be achieved. Once the school sees the benefits, they may welcome the shadow teacher to stay longer.

Another powerful way to quickly build rapport with the teacher is a teacher's home visit, which is not common in many countries. Speak to your setting and see what they can offer your child.

DOI: 10.4324/9781003355267-3

Finally, the section emphasises the importance of one-on-one time with the teacher in school and providing support at various times, including before and after class, after-school programs, and during school breaks.

Overall, this section provides practical examples for teachers to support their students with SM both in and outside of school. It highlights the importance of building rapport, easing transitions, and providing support at various settings and times to help the child progress toward recovery.

## Letter to Teaching Staff

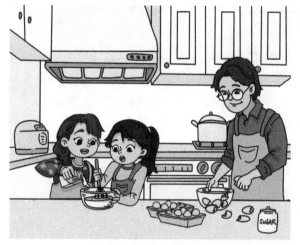

Happy and talkative at home

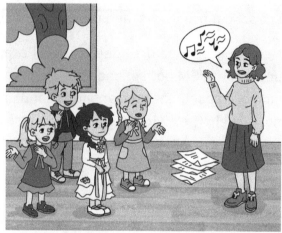

Silent and anxious at school

Dear _____,

We would like to introduce our daughter, Amy, who is a bright and sweet girl. She loves to dance, sing, ice skate, swim, go horseback riding, and have playdates with her friends. Amy is a chatterbox at home and talks freely with family. However, she gets nervous and has difficulties getting her words out in school. This is due to a type of childhood anxiety disorder called selective mutism (SM). SM is a fear of speaking, but it can be overcome with the proper support in place. Amy needs your help to communicate at school. Please see the attached videos of Amy talking with family and friends at home and in the park. Below are some recommendations from the SM specialist on how to interact with Amy in school.

1. **Keep her busy:** Let Amy help with things that she is capable of, such as passing and collecting class materials, organising the bookshelf, and accompanying other students to the bathroom or nurse's office.
2. **Graded question sequence:** Start with easier "Yes/No" questions, which can be answered non-verbally, then move on to forced-choice questions. Avoid asking the more difficult open-ended questions.

   a. Yes/no question: Do you like dogs? This type of question can be answered by nodding/shaking your head.
   b. Forced-choice question: Do you like dogs or rabbits?
   c. Closed questions (single words, then phrases): Which planet has rings? Where is Big Ben?
   d. Open-ended question: What kind of animals do you like? What did you do during the weekend?

3. **Five-second waiting rule:** Wait for five seconds for Amy to answer a question. If there is no response after five seconds, rephrase it as an easier question (see above). If there is still no response, make a friendly comment and move on.
4. **Greet and chat:** Please do greet and chat with Amy, but do not expect Amy to respond verbally. She may use gestures, such as nodding, shaking her head, and pointing. She may also be able to talk or whisper to her friends, write, and draw pictures. Amy has difficulties initiating conversations, so please try to anticipate her needs and check that she understands her work.
5. **Lunch with teachers:** Letting Amy and her talking buddy have lunch with a teacher on a regular basis can be very helpful. She may start to talk when she is away from the large group of classmates.
6. **Rehearsal:** Let Amy know the class questions/group assignments at least one day in advance. This will give her more time to prepare and rehearse her answers at home.
7. **Be patient:** Recognise small progress. It is important not to make a big fuss when Amy starts to talk. Keep the conversation going as usual and simply tell her, "Thanks for sharing that with me!" or "That's a good idea".
8. **Communication book:** Amy keeps a journal at home where she writes down new things she wants to share or questions she wants to ask. Please ask her to show you, then answer the questions and write/ask new questions.

Amy will initially answer you through talking buddy or by nodding. Drawing Amy into the conversation this way will build a bond between Amy and the teacher and ease her into spoken dialogue.

## Tips and Tricks

- This letter is an example to inspire parents to write a heart-to-heart letter to school officials.
- Parents can also attach videos showing that a child can speak, sing, dance, and run at home and in the community when they are not anxious. These videos will motivate the school staff to help children to reach their best.

## Teachers Are the No. 3 Essential Component in SM Recovery Journey

A teacher's influence lasts for eternity; one can never predict where their impact ends. With teachers participating, it makes the intervention successful, and effects last a lifetime. Table 3.1 summarises the strategies for use, the challenges children with SM face, and the support teachers and staff can provide in their recovery journey. The information in this table can be utilised as supplemental material for an Individualised Education Plan (IEP) to identify challenges and request support. Readers can follow the pictures and sections indicated to read more.

**TABLE 3.1  Teacher/staff support in the child's SM recovery journey**

| No. | Category | Examples of activities | | |
|-----|----------|------------------------|---|---|
| 1 | **School staff work –** Study SM strategies, build up intervention plan with SM treating professional, understand "Dos and don'ts for children" (Part 2, 3) | Parents demonstrate strategies to teachers | Counsellor trains teacher about SM strategies | Communication book |
| 2 | **Strategies in school –** Offer talking opportunity (Part 3, 4) | Observe butterflies with buddies | Be a helper in Holiday party | Presentation in moving up day |
| 3 | **Strategies in school –** Keep the child busy, create talking opportunity (Part 3, 4) | Teacher's helper | Subject helper | Teacher's shadow |
| 4 | **Strategies in school –** one-on-one with teacher (Part 3) | One-on-one with teacher in a private room | One-on-one with teacher and a buddy in a private room | One-on-one with teacher in the classroom |
| 5 | **Strategies in school –** Small group with a buddy Sit next to a buddy; Rotate NEW classmate to the group ONE by ONE; Rotate talking buddy once talking to a new person established (Part 3) | Small group with teacher in the cafeteria | Small group in a classroom corner | Small group practice before Gym class |
| 6 | **Strategies in school –** Present to the whole class (Part 3,4) | Talent show in front of the class | Presentation to the class | Show and tell in the classroom |

(Continued)

**TABLE 3.1** (Continued)

| No. | Category | Examples of activities | | |
|---|---|---|---|---|
| 7 | **Counsellor work** (Part 3, 4) | One-on-one/small group in a private room | Assigned jobs – provide talking opportunity | Walkie-talkie under desk – using a device |
| 8 | **Challenges –** Health issues and social skills (Part 4) | Bathroom, lunch, report health issues | Bully | Alone in recess, break, and discussion time |
| 9 | **Challenges –** Academic: Fail in all subjects that require communication (Part 4) | Music – not able to sing <br>Art – cannot tell missing materials | Math – unable to answer questions or ask for help <br>Science – cannot answer questions even after raising hand | Cannot express or opinions in oral exams <br>Library – cannot participate in group story discussion |
| 10 | **Support in school** (Part 3) | Private tour before school starts | Private tour before school ends (moving up day) | Private tour before Back to School Night |

(Continued)

**TABLE 3.1** (Continued)

| No. | Category | Examples of activities | | |
|-----|----------|------------------------|---|---|
| 11 | **Support outside of school** (Part 3) | Home visit | Meet in public | Communicate by text, video, voice message, facetime |

# Dos and Don'ts List for Teachers

**Do**

1. Understanding SM is an anxiety disorder, not a personal choice. Educate other students about SM, so they can become the child's buddies and include the child in their group activities.

2. Greet and chat with the child in a friendly manner without expecting or demanding a verbal response.

3. Take the pressure of speaking off the child and let the child know in private that they may talk when they are ready; use a soft voice as children with SM are easily intimidated.

4. Accept all forms of communication at first. Encourage the child to communicate using whatever they are comfortable with, such as gestures, pointing, nodding, whispering, using props and puppets, and so on.

5. Accommodate the child for essential needs in daily life, e.g., no need to request verbally for using the restroom, eating, drinking, and first aid.

6. Pair the child with a buddy for classwork and activities. Make the child feel included and welcomed.

7. Pay attention to the child's body language for anxiety levels – the less animated and mobile they are, the more anxious they feel. If the child doesn't respond to you, it's not because she is naughty/defiant. She is unable to.

8. Five-second rule. Wait for five seconds for the child to think and prepare their answers.

9. Know the difficulty level for the asked questions, i.e., yes/no, choice, and direct.

10. Communicate with parents about the child's behaviour in school. Discuss any other issues the child has that may cause them concern or increase their anxiety.

11. Team up with parents, professionals, and school psychologist. Understand the intervention plan and communicate the progress. Learn different SM strategies and implement them as consistently as possible.

12. Use parents, siblings, talking buddies, or friends to help the child get comfortable talking in front of you and eventually talk to you.

13. One-on-one time with the child in a private space to build rapport. Parents will provide video/audio of the child talking outside of school. Play video/audio recording with the child for voice exposure and desensitisation.

14. Take small and gradual steps to help the child expand their talking circle. Include new children and adults, one person at a time, and gradually increase the

communication load from non-verbal communication (gesture) to familiar rote-learned speech (reading, counting, fixed language in games, etc.), single words, and sentences.

15. Expect the same good behaviour for the SM child as any other child.
16. Enlist the child as a teacher's helper. Give the child tasks which may not require verbal communication.
17. Provide support such as pairing the child with a buddy to give them the confidence to do things themselves; engage and include the child in group activities by accepting all forms of communication. Stay positive even when progress seems slow, and have a backup plan in case the child is overwhelmed by a new challenge.
18. Providing observations/videos will help give the treating professional and parents a clearer picture. For example, observe if the child can eat and use the bathroom in school, has any academic challenges, or experiences difficulties in class/group participation.
19. Give labelled praise for verbal and non-verbal interactions, e.g., "Good job for telling/showing me…".

1. Ignore the child.
2. Try to force, coax, or beg the child to talk.
3. Pressure the child to speak, put him in the spotlight, or say, "you're very quiet".
4. Get upset or take it personally if the child does not respond to you.
5. Congratulate the child when you first hear the child speaking. Do respond naturally.
6. Enable the child to become dependent on non-verbal communication.
7. Approach the child without understanding their condition and action plan.
8. Get discouraged if progress seems slow or stalled.
9. Guess what the child wants by mind-reading.

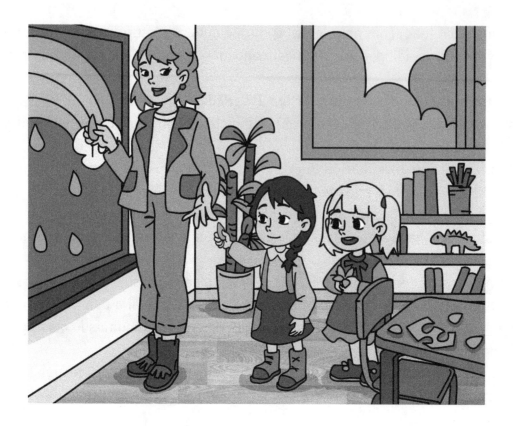

## Visiting New School before the New Year/Term/Semester

As part of the school's helping plan, Amy and her mom could choose to visit the new school a few times before the fall semester began. Today, Amy and her mom invited Amy's talking buddy Sofie to meet their new teacher Ms. Bo. Ms. Bo invited the girls to set up the classroom together. Before getting to work, Ms. Bo played a playdate video that showed Amy and Sofie shopping for stationery supplies in a local shop together. Both Amy and Sofie's voices could be clearly heard. Ms. Bo commented on the video with light-hearted remarks.

She then left the girls to do some designing and cutting and was pleased to listen to them chatting together.

Now it was time to decorate the whiteboard. "Amy, please pass a raindrop sticker to me. Is this a good spot to place it?" Ms. Bo asked. Amy handed the sticker to Ms. Bo and nodded her head. "Do you want to place it higher or lower?" Ms. Bo continued asking. Amy thought for a few seconds and said, "A bit higher". "What should we place on the board next, a rainbow or a tree sticker?" Ms. Bo asked while placing the raindrop sticker without looking at Amy directly. "Rainbow!" Amy answered loudly.

## Tips and Tricks

- Prepare the child for the transition to a new school in advance. Help the child think of the move as a fresh start and make it a positive experience. If you can, visit the new teacher and classroom during the summer break to get familiarised.
- The teacher should treat the SM child the same way as other children, except for the part where they may not talk. Setting a positive tone in the classroom that allows children to express themselves differently, either verbally or non-verbally, will alleviate the talking pressure and encourage participation.
- To ease SM child's transition into a new school, find a supportive adult/ keyworker to help the child settle initial difficulties in school and keep open communication with parents.
- Invite along a child's sibling or talking buddy as appropriate. Parents, siblings, or talking buddies can provide a talking bridge to facilitate conversations with the new teacher (see page 86).

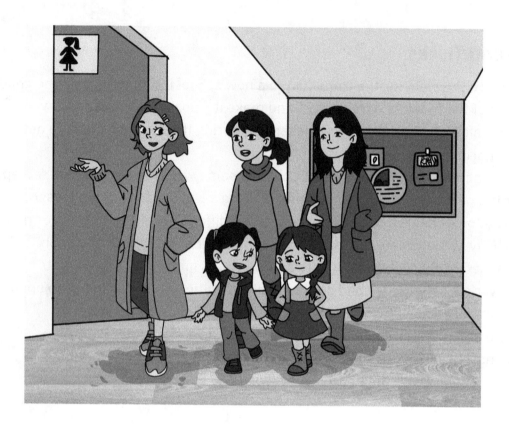

## Back to School Night

Amy and her mom offered Jada and her mom a ride to Back to School Night. They were the first group arriving at school when it was still quiet and less crowded. As Amy walked around the school, Ms. Kerri showed them various school facilities, such as the nurse's office, main office, gym, cafeteria, and restrooms. She also showed them where the pencil sharpener, books, paper, and other supplies were located in the homeroom. They also met with and were introduced to other teachers during their tour.

While parents were meeting with teachers, Amy, Jada, and a few classmates played a game that Amy had brought. Amy showed and whispered to Jada how to play the game. Then Jada explained to others, repeating what Amy had told her.

Amy, Jada, and their moms checked out all the important spots, such as the bathroom, cafeteria, and nurse's office in the building one more time before heading home.

## Tips and Tricks

- If the child has already had a private tour of the school before school starts, they can be the teacher's helpers at "Back to School Night". The child can show classmates where things are.
- On the private tour and Back to School Night, the child comes with a buddy to whom the child talks outside of school. This buddy will act as a talking bridge connecting the child with the teacher and classmates: the child has conversations with the talking buddy in the presence of others, which leads to the talking buddy acting as a go-between, i.e., the child answers or asks questions via the talking buddy in preparation for talking to others directly.
- "The first one to arrive and the last one to leave" gives more opportunities to meet other parents, share about SM, set up playdates and find out about the after-school programs that classmates attend.

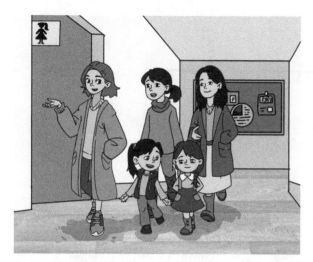 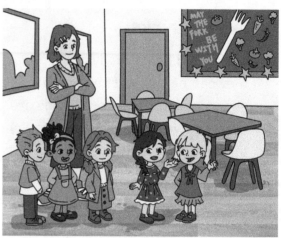

## Private Tour (Left) and Moving up Day (Right) before School Year End

Amy graduated from 1st grade and was looking forward to starting her 2nd grade at a new school. Amy's mom requested a private tour of the school before the school year ended. She also asked if Amy's talking buddy Sofie could be in the same class with Amy to increase Amy's comfort level.

Amy went on a private tour with her current 1st-grade teacher Ms. Kerri and her talking buddy Sofie. During the private tour, along with Sofie's voice "hi", Amy was able to greet the teachers they met in the hallway, though sometimes the teachers hardly heard Amy's voice. They stopped by the nurse's office, played games in the counsellor's room, and visited their new classroom. They walked around the school to get familiarised with various facilities, i.e., the nurse's office, main office, gymnasium, cafeteria, library, and restrooms. Amy's new teacher also went over the classroom layout, such as where the books, sharpeners, paper, and supplies were. Amy's voice was much louder when they left the school.

On moving up day (orientation), Amy was excited that she and Sofie were asked to be the teacher's helpers since they had a private tour before. Amy helped her peers find their seats, showed them where the books, pencil sharpeners, and bathrooms were located, and pointed to the classroom calendar with the classroom routine. When her new teacher asked the class questions, Amy told Sofie what she wanted to say, then Sofie spoke out for her.

## Tips and Tricks

- The new teacher can join the private tour and set up tasks that will help the child interact with their peers later, such as showing classmates where the books are and accompanying them to the bathroom.
- The result of the private tour (visiting the school and classroom, meeting the teachers, etc.) can drastically reduce discomfort on orientation day and promote confidence in communicating with classmates in different forms, such as pointing and talking via talking buddy. It is worthwhile to prepare ahead.
- The child may not respond to spontaneous questions from a classmate. If standing close by, the talking buddy or teacher can repeat or rephrase the questions to a yes/no, or a choice question.

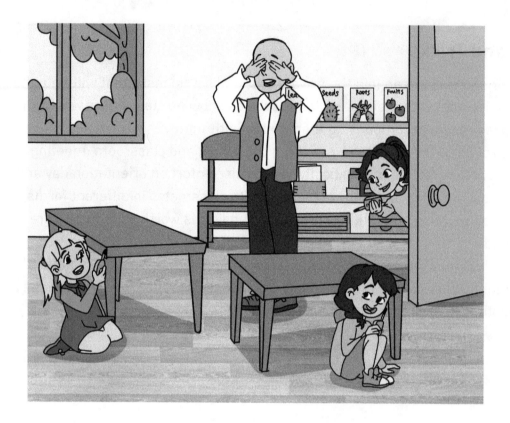

## Private Time with Counsellor and Buddy

As part of her IEP plan, Amy and her talking buddy, Sofie, would meet Mr. Alex, the counsellor, at his office for half an hour once a week. Before meeting Mr. Alex, Amy had been communicating with her teachers and classmates using text messages, the smartwatch, a talking album, the communication notebook, and a talking puppy that was a recording device. Mr. Alex aimed to help Amy speak verbally in his office before moving their conversations into the classroom and other parts of the school, such as the cafeteria and the playground.

Before starting a fun game, Mr. Alex would first play a voice recording of Amy and Sofie. Then he gave each girl a walkie-talkie and told them to hide and he would try to find them. Amy loved to play hide and seek. She talked excitedly to Sofie through the walkie-talkie about where Mr. Alex was. When Mr. Alex asked, "Is anybody behind the door or under the chair?" Amy and Sofie would use the walkie-talkie to say "nope" to trick him and then quietly move to another hiding spot.

Amy liked spending time in Mr. Alex's office because they would play fun games, such as hide and seek and treasure hunt. She also liked Mr. Alex's funny jokes and stories. Amy quickly opened up to Mr. Alex, especially when Sofie was there with her.

Once Amy talked to Mr. Alex, they began moving their activities outside the office.

## Tips and Tricks

- Voice recording is a very helpful step toward SM recovery as it desensitises the child to the sound of their own voice and being overheard. For the child, allowing others to hear their voice recording is a stepping stone to speaking face to face.
- Teacher can build rapport with the child through fun games and activities, such as guessing games, hide-and-seeking objects, treasure hunts, and quizzes using voice recordings. Play a voice recording of the child at the beginning of the session and use graded questioning throughout (see page 76).

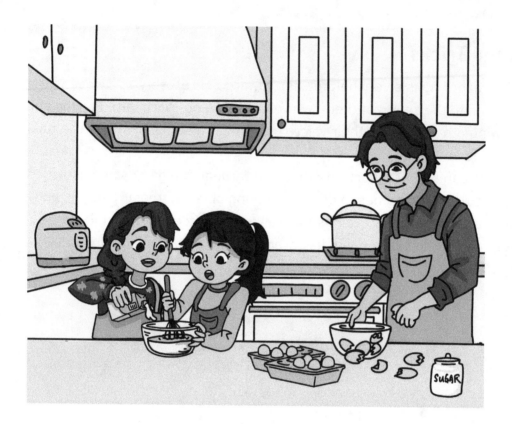

## Teacher's Home Visit

Amy was excited about the home visit from her teacher Ms. Lana, and wanted to make cookies for her. Amy invited her talking buddy Jada to help her. They cracked eggs, poured flour, and added milk and butter into the bowl. As they discussed the ingredients and steps and passed the items, the challenge came, either they had too much water or too much flour. The dough got bigger and bigger each time they added more water or flour. "Where is the measuring cup?" Amy's dad had to step in before their dough got out of control. The girls giggled and went to look for a measuring cup.

## Tips and Tricks

- A home visit by a current or new teacher can be very effective in helping SM children talk in school. Teachers' time commitment may pay off significantly since it will shorten the school intervention period. Ask if this is an option at your school.
- The main goal is to build rapport and accelerate the child's social comfort through fun activities with no pressure to talk. Teachers need to be sensitive and only gradually enter the child's personal space, especially during the initial home visit.
- Before the teacher arrives, engage the child in a fun and exciting game/ activity that leads to spontaneous conversations.
- One parent or a friend keeps playing and talking with the child after the teacher arrives. The other parent can welcome the teacher and perhaps offer them a drink while the child gets used to their presence.
- If only one parent is available for teacher visits, this parent should play games, bake, or have the child's favourite activities with the child before the teacher comes. When the teacher arrives, the parent and the teacher can have a drink and chat on one side of the room. At the same time, the parent chats with the child, to help the child continue talking with the teacher present. The teacher gradually interacts with the child.

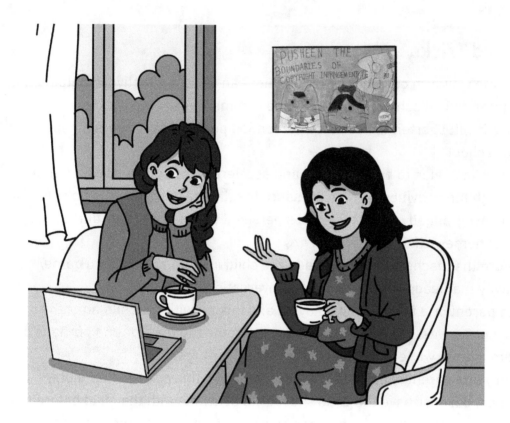

## Teacher's Arrival

When Ms. Lana arrived, she came by and waved hello to the baking crew in the kitchen, then went to chat with Mom in the living room. Ms. Lana sat in a position where she could hear Amy without directly seeing her. Amy was too occupied with her baking task to pay attention to Ms. Lana. She continued working and talking normally with Jada and Dad.

Mom showed Ms. Lana a family gathering video that had Amy's voice clearly recorded. The video was played at a volume loud enough that Amy could hear it from the kitchen. Mom and Ms. Lana later walked into the kitchen but kept a distance from Amy. Ms. Lana avoided making direct eye contact or talking to Amy. She pretended to be busy checking out plants in the garden and asking Mom about them. As Amy continued talking in the presence of Ms. Lana, Ms. Lana walked closer to the counter to check out the cookie dough.

Dad brought Ms. Lana into the conversation. Ms Lana chatted to Dad and complimented the girls on their baking. Once Amy was talking easily to Dad, only a short distance from Ms. Lana, he made an excuse to leave the kitchen Mom could take over now!

## Tips and Tricks

- If children are anxious about the teacher's visit, parents can reassure them that they will make sure the child has a good time. Explain that the teacher is just visiting to see how fun their home life is and make a casual suggestion of ways to welcome a guest, e.g., wave hello, offer a cup of water, give a tour of their room, show the teacher their favourite toy, share a fun video, etc.
- Voice exposure is useful to prepare children for talking directly to others and takes three forms: a) Child is happy to share an audio or video recording which allows their voice to be heard; b) Child has a conversation with family or friends in the presence of others; c) Child says something to family or a friend which they want to be passed on to someone else.

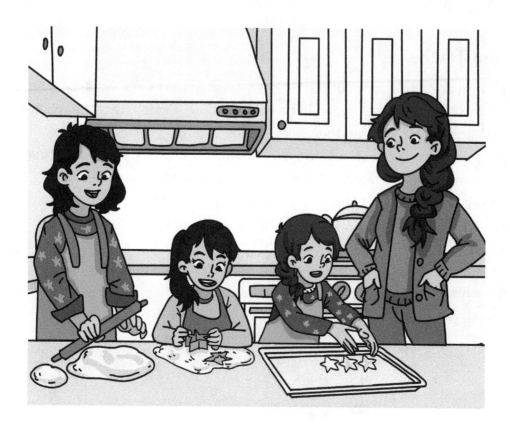

## Teacher Participates in Child's Work/Activity

Amy and Jada were busy using a cookie cutter to cut cookies. "You cut them out; I'll put them on the baking tray", said Amy. Mom and Ms. Lana watched from the side. Ms. Lana made friendly comments about cookies and asked rhetorical questions which needed no answer. "I love cookies in a star shape. They look fantastic, don't they?" Amy nodded in agreement. Mom helped Amy start talking again by asking Amy a choice question, "How many batches of cookies are we going to make, Amy, one or two?" "Two!" Jada answered, forgetting that she should let Amy try to answer for herself. "Maybe three, maybe more", Amy said with a smile. "Your mom told me that you guys would make only one batch of cookies", said Ms. Lana. The girls then went on explaining how the cookie dough got bigger and bigger, so now they'd got enough for several batches. Ms. Lana was surprised to hear Amy talking but refrained from showing it. She carried on normally as if Amy had always spoken to her. She moved over to the table to count the stars. Seeing Amy comfortably speaking in front of Ms. Lana, Amy's mom went to preheat the oven.

## Tips and Tricks

- Inform the child of the date and time of a home visit in advance, and invite them to plan activities they would like to do with the teacher, e.g., playing card games, making handicrafts, baking cookies, etc.
- If possible and appropriate, invite a friend that the child enjoys talking to.
- If the child is happily engaged in an activity, the teacher or new person can enter the room and first observe from the side, then gradually move closer to the child, and finally join in the activity. If the child speaks to family or friends, as in this example, try to engage with the child at a distance and then slide in.
- The parent facilitates conversation and withdraws after the child talks comfortably in front of the teacher (sliding-out).
- The teacher uses commentary style talk in the beginning (see page 60). If the child looks relaxed, the teacher can gradually ask questions in a sequence of "yes/no".

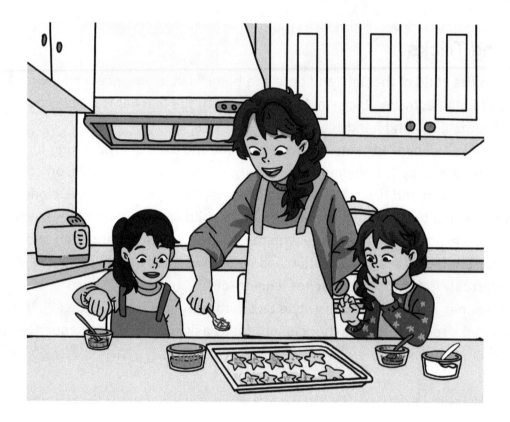

## Teacher and Child Decorating Cookies Together

"Ding!" the oven went off. Amy and Jada jumped up and shouted with joy, "Yay, our cookies are done!" While they were waiting for the cookies to cool down, Ms. Lana, Amy, and Jada got the icing and toppings ready. "I want the green icing". Jada grabbed the green container. Left with blue and red containers, Ms. Lana asked Amy, "Would you like the blue or red icing?" Amy said without hesitation, "Red, please!"

Amy, Jada, and Ms. Lana decorated the cookies with the colour in front of them. When Amy was busy licking delicious sprinkles off her finger, Ms. Lana joked, "Amy! There won't be enough left for the cookies!"

The decorated cookies looked so nice that they took them to school to share with classmates. In addition, they wanted to show a video of how to make cookies in their show and tell. Ms. Lana suggested that Jada could do the "tell" while Amy did the "Show". So, on the last batch, Jada recorded while Amy was making. They also rehearsed with mom the possible questions their classmates might ask, such as "What flavours are the cookies?" "Can I have two?"

## Tips and Tricks

- A home visit can help the teacher learn more about the child and see first-hand how the child is able to communicate verbally when different strategies are applied, such as commentary style talk/Sportscaster (page 60), sliding-in and out (pages 57, 62, 64), voice-exposure (pages 13, 95), graded questioning (page 76)
- Once the teacher and the child talk at home, the teacher can serve as a talking bridge between the child and others, bringing the child's voice into school. They can also take a 'keyworker' role and organise short sessions to help the child generalise their talking to other adults and children.

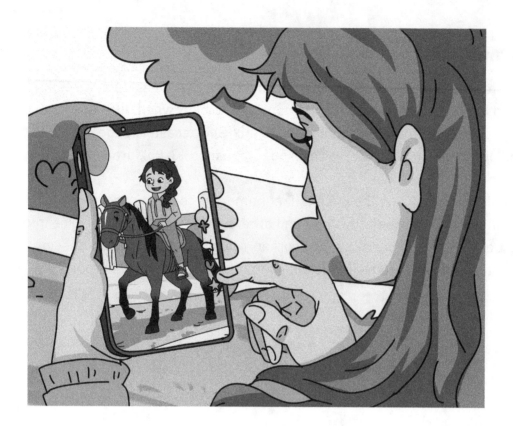

## Rapport Building with Teachers after School and on School Break

When school was out for the summer break, Amy and her Social Studies teacher, Ms. Sandy, had agreed to exchange text messages with videos of themselves.

Today, Amy went to ride her horse in the barn. She was excited to share her horse-riding video with Ms. Sandy. After receiving and watching Amy's video, Ms. Sandy sent Amy voice messages asking her questions about her horse, "What's the name of your horse? Is it a girl or a boy? How much does it weigh?" Amy's mom helped Amy practise answering Ms. Sandy's questions before sending voice messages back. Amy told Ms. Sandy, "My horse's name is Stella. She's a girl and weighs 1,500 lbs. She is my good friend and likes me to brush the hair on her legs". Ms. Sandy was surprised but happy to hear Amy's voice. She sent back a video of her long-haired puppy. Amy asked questions about the puppy, "What's his name? He looks like a 'lion' dog. With so much hair covering his eyes, can he see what's in front of him?"

Amy and Ms. Sandy also had a weekly reading session online via webcam. They would read a story together or chat that Amy had first practised at home. Then Ms. Sandy would ask a few questions about the story, and Amy's mom would help Amy rehearse the answers ahead of time. They also met once in the park. They watched Amy's playdate videos at first, then played a ball-throwing game while naming different fruits.

Amy and Ms. Sandy had built a good rapport during the summer break. When the school reopened in September, they moved their video-watching and Q&A sessions into school. Ms. Sandy then invited other teachers and classmates, one at a time to these sessions. They first watched a video with Amy's voice clearly recorded, then either had Q&A or played a fun game that led to verbal communication.

## Tips and Tricks

- See if your school can offer any opportunities to stay connected and build rapport with teachers when school is out, e.g., exchanging videos, sending voice messages, meeting online via webcam.

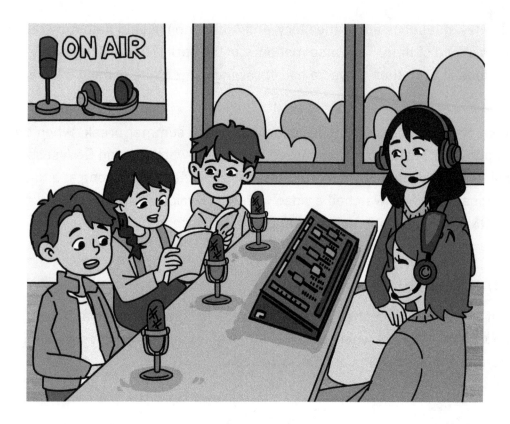

## Little Broadcaster – Meeting Teacher outside of School

Today, Amy's mom invited Amy's teacher, Ms. Kerri, and her two sons to the radio station. "Amy, please show William and Henry how to set up the microphone", Mom said, "Okay, let's go through today's schedule. We are going to read books, sing a song, and...". Amy's mom paused and looked at Amy, and Amy continued, "tell jokes and accept audience calls before the weather forecast".

Ms. Kerri was surprised to see Amy speak so confidently and spontaneously. She'd only said a few words to her at school. But she tried to act as she normally would and carried on the conversation. She asked Amy, "What do you like best, reporting, forecasting, or reading stories?... How many classmates have been invited to the radio station?... What is next week's topic?" Amy answered all her questions without needing any help. For the rest of the term, Ms. Kerri let Amy hand out invitations she had prepped at home to other classmates whom Amy had never spoken to in school, further expanding Amy's talking circle.

## Tips and Tricks

- Teacher and child can meet outside of school, in an informal setting to build rapport. Try to meet in a place where the child is most comfortable, such as home or a place they often visit. Join in an activity that the child is interested in and good at in order to help the child open up quickly.

- Once the child talks to the teacher spontaneously outside of school, they can move the conversation into school. First, in a private room, they could play the child's video together to allow the child's voice to be heard. Then repeat an aspect of the outside activity which the child is already familiar with and move into general conversation. Add new people one by one into the room and repeat the same exercise.

- It may not be possible to arrange a home visit but speak with the school and find out what alternatives might be on offer.

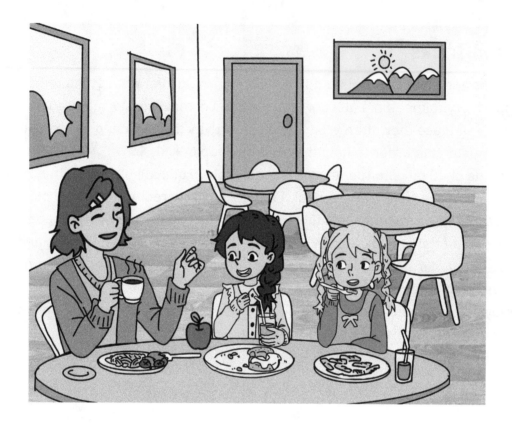

## Private Time with Teacher/Classmate in the School Cafeteria

The school has started a few months now. Even though Amy had spoken to Ms. Kerri at the evening event before school started, she had yet to talk to her during school time. Seeing Amy progressing nicely with her classmates at lunchtime, Amy's mom suggested that Ms. Kerri eat lunch with Amy and Sam.

Ms. Kerri met Amy and Sam in the school cafeteria. They sat at a table in the corner. Amy and Sam whispered to each other as they ate. Seeing the apples on her plate, Amy asked Sam, "Who does eating an apple a day keep away?" Sam guessed, "Dog? Cat? Bunny?..." "No, silly!" they started giggling. "I know", said Ms. Kerri, "Eating an apple a day keeps the doctor away". Amy smiled and nodded. Ms. Kerri joined their conversation. "And eating an onion a day keeps whom away?" Sam joked, "A bug? A worm?" Amy shook her head and said, "Eating an onion a day keeps everyone away!" Although Amy said it to Sam, her voice was loud enough for Ms. Kerri to hear. After a few rounds of jokes and games, Amy was able to respond to Ms. Kerri directly.

## Tips and Tricks

- Build rapport by having one-on-one time with the teacher in a separate space or a corner of the room.
- Child's talking buddy can act as a bridge connecting the child and the new person.
- Parents can help the child practise telling funny jokes at home to increase their confidence in telling jokes outside.

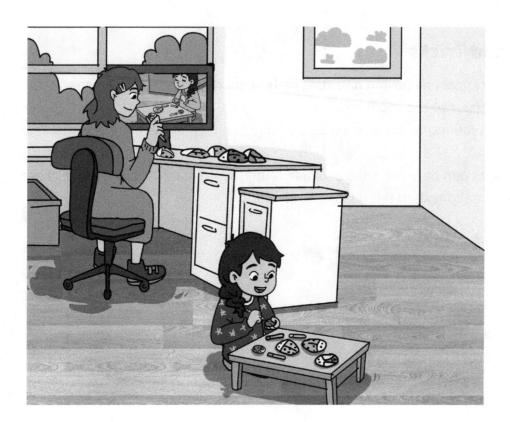

## Painting with Teacher – One-on-One Time in a Private Room

Amy liked art work, and painting stones was one of her favourite activities. Mom asked Amy to teach her how to paint a stone step by step at home. Amy told Mom, "First, you need to draw a ladybug. Then you paint its wings in a colour you like, and don't forget to add dots!" With Amy's permission, Mom recorded the whole activity and shared it with Amy's teacher, Ms. Kerri.

At school, Ms. Kerri invited Amy to paint stones in her office. While Amy was painting her stones, Ms. Kerri was also doing the same thing by playing and following the steps mentioned in Amy's video. Ms. Kerri talked to herself, "This is fun! I have ladybugs in blue, red, and yellow. Now, did I forget anything? Oh, yes, I forgot to add dots!" Amy turned around to check out what Ms. Kerri was doing. Then Ms. Kerri asked, "Amy, do you have a black colour?" Amy responded by nodding. "How many dots should I add to each ladybug's wings? 8 or 10?" said Ms. Kerri. Amy replied, "10". Ms. Kerri was over the moon this was the first time Amy had spoken to her without her talking buddy present. But she didn't remark on it. She simply replied, "OK, 10 dots coming up!"

## Tips and Tricks

- One-on-one with the teacher in a private space helps build a good rapport with the child, which is essential for further support and progress in school.
- Parents make it a habit of voice-recording or videotaping the child. Tell the child that it is just for fun and a great way to show others how much fun she has at home. These clips can be short and casual, but the child's voice should be heard clearly, e.g., reading a storybook, explaining the rules of a board game, or singing a song learned in school. If the child seems concerned, reassure them that other people know they can talk at home and are happy to wait until the child is ready to talk to them too.
- For the purpose of desensitisation, the teacher plays these recordings/videos with the child in a private space, comments using commentary style talk, and accepts all forms of communication from the child. Once the child is actively engaged in an activity, questions are gradually introduced using the graded question sequence on page 76.
- The video sent to teachers can be the child talking to family, friends, and classmates. With the child's permission, the teacher may like to use academic-related videos, such as explaining the butterfly life cycle in science class or reading a book in language class. The teacher can, with the child's consent, progressively play these videos in private, small groups or in front of the class, so the child would gradually accept her voice being exposed to the public (graded exposure) The classmates may start to ask questions about the videos, therefore providing a talking opportunity.
- Self-modelling is a technique where a video or audio recording of a child speaking in a comfortable environment is played back to the child in an environment where they may feel uncomfortable or hesitant to speak. By seeing and hearing themselves speak confidently in a similar setting, the child can become more comfortable and confident in their ability to communicate effectively in that environment.

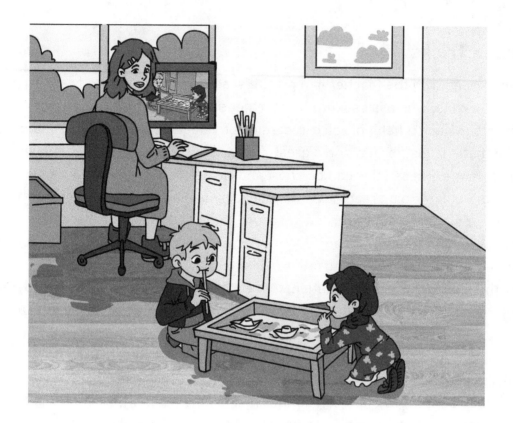

## Racing Boats – With Teacher and Talking Buddy in a Private Room

Ms. Kerri invited Amy and James, Amy's talking buddy, to her office to play the boat racing game. Amy and James played the same game at Amy's house the day before. Amy's mom recorded it and shared it with Ms. Kerri. Ms. Kerri sat in front of her desk, watching the video while Amy and James played the game a short distance away. Amy could hear her voice and was a bit nervous about Ms. Kerri's reaction, but her game helped to distract her. "Looks like Amy's boat is faster". Ms. Kerri commented from her desk. "No, I don't think so, Ms. Kerri", James said. "It is! I'm going to win this time", Amy spoke loudly and clearly in front of Ms. Kerri. "This looks so much fun! You don't mind if I join you guys, do you?" Ms. Kerri asked as she knelt down with them. Amy nodded excitedly. "I'll make a boat for you". Amy got up to get a piece of paper.

## Tips and Tricks

- A competitive and fun game can get the child excited and engaged, leading to a spontaneous speech where the child initiates conversation. The adult can choose appropriate activities and materials for the child to fully engage at a comfortable pace, based on the child's likes and interests. Inviting a talking buddy to join the game helps accelerate speech.
- To help the child desensitise, the teacher plays a recording or a video with the child's voice before the game. Teacher can start as an observer on the side, move closer to the game, and finally join in the game.
- Working towards spontaneous speech, the teacher can comment on the game, ask rhetorical questions, then ask yes/no or choice questions. It takes time for the child to respond, first with gestures, then single words, phrases and sentences, and lastly, spontaneous comments. This won't happen immediately. It will take time and patience.
- Children often find it easier to speak to a new person when there is some distance between them.
- If free play is not successful in eliciting spontaneous speech, play games where the children take turns to ask questions, give clues, or issue instructions. They will be practising initiating conversation in a game before they do it spontaneously.

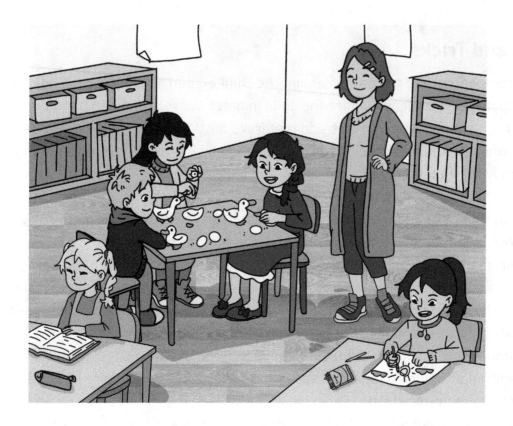

## Playing in a Small Group at the Classroom Corner

Amy had been able to talk comfortably to Ms. Kerri and her talking buddies, Rosa and James, in Ms. Kerri's office. It was time to move their activities into the classroom! Ms. Kerri put Amy, Rosa, and James in the same group during the free-play time. Their table was placed in the classroom corner to draw less attention from others.

While Amy, Rosa, and James were chatting and making clay ducks, other classmates were nearby busy with their activities, but they could hear Amy's voice. Occasionally, Ms. Kerri and a few classmates passed by the table or watched them playing clay. "Can I join you? What are you making? Are you making ducks or geese?" When their classmates asked questions, Rosa and James answered unless the question was explicitly directed at Amy. If Amy could not respond, they either repeated/rephrased the question or walked close to Amy and said, "tell me".

"Amy, your duck looks like a rooster, cock-a-doodle-do". Ms. Kerri joked while everyone was busy with their clay creations. Amy quickly responded, "Then Rosa's looks like a cat. Meow, meow! And James' looks like a dog, woof, woof!" Everyone laughed and giggled because they all knew Rosa loved cats and James loved dogs.

## Tips and Tricks

- It is more likely that young children will make sounds of joy/excitement/ animal noises if engaged in enjoyable play. Releasing the voice through play may lead to words and sentences.
- For group/class discussion, teacher puts the child with classmates they have spoken to in the same group. Child can choose to answer through their talking buddy, read the answer in front of the group/class, or answer directly without anyone's support.
- Teacher makes light-hearted jokes or fun comments about the activity to help the child relax and engage in conversation. Once the teacher has established a good rapport and talked with the child one-on-one, the teacher can act as a bridge to connect the child with his/her classmates.
- To expand the circle of talking buddies, a new non-talking-buddy classmate will be assigned to the table, and classmates rotation gives the child opportunities to speak to everyone in the classroom.

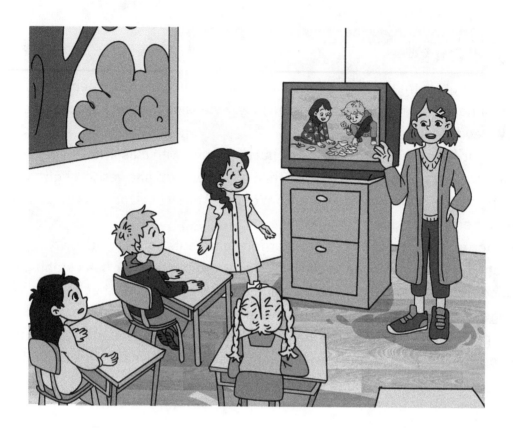

## Circle Time/Presentation in Front of the Class

Amy had allowed Ms. Kerri and a group of her classmates to hear her voice. Now, it was time to let the whole class hear her. During today's circle time and with Amy's permission, Ms. Kerri played a video of Amy and James' playdate in the park. They picked up fallen leaves, piled them up, stomped on them, and threw them in the air while shouting, "Raining, falling, flying...". They were having such a great time. Everyone smiled while watching the video.

Ms. Kerri invited Amy to talk briefly about her playdate using "when, where, who, and what" – the structure that all the class used for their news. Amy read from her notes. She had practised saying these lines at home and had rehearsed with Ms. Kerri in advance. Then it was Q&A time with classmates. Amy could answer some questions using adequate volume. For other questions, Ms. Kerri helped by answering the first part of the sentence and letting Amy finish the rest, e.g., Ms. Kerri started, "Amy, you picked up leaves and..." "A pine cone". Amy answered.

## Tips and Tricks

- Using a two-way/home-school communication book, the teacher tells the child and parents circle time topics in advance and discusses non-verbal/verbal participation options to include the child. The teacher assures the child that they will only talk about the topic and questions rehearsed and nothing beyond that.
- To reduce the anxiety and pressure of talking, the child can pre-record what they want to say at home and play the video during circle time.
- The child rehearses and practises talking for circle time with the teacher, their talking buddies, or parents before presenting in front of the whole class.
- Good readers find reading aloud easier than free conversation, so this, or something they have learned off by heart, is best for their first presentation.
- Have a backup plan just in case the child is too overwhelmed to speak, e.g., have the child's buddy who was in the video co-present.

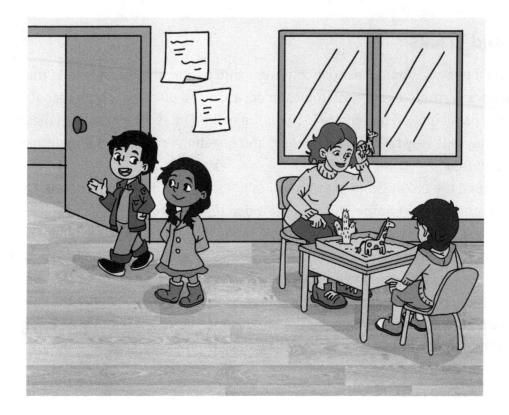

## One-on-One Time with the Teacher between Classes

All her classmates were attending the art class except Ms. Cookie and Amy.

They stayed behind to spend one-on-one time during the 5-minute class transition period. Ms. Cookie sometimes played videos or audios shared by Amy's parents. Together, they watched/listened to these clips with Amy's voice clearly recorded. Ms. Cookie would make light-hearted comments. Afterwards, and as Amy got more and more comfortable, Ms. Cookie would start to ask graded questions and play simple turn-taking games with her. For example, Ms. Cookie would roll a ball to Amy and say an animal's name, "tiger", and Amy would roll the ball back to her while saying "gorilla".

Amy gradually built rapport with Ms. Cookie and talked to her during one-on-one time. Ms. Cookie then invited other classmates one by one to join them in doing the same exercise. First, they played videos/audios to make Amy's voice heard. Then they played a game that required simple speech, e.g., Duck, Duck, Goose!, Uno, etc.

## Tips and Tricks

- Teachers have busy schedules, making it difficult to find one-on-one time with children. It is important to be creative and make each private session short yet effective.
- Some good time slots to hold mini-sessions with teachers are before/after school, recess, lunch, and between classes. Some teachers are willing to meet children outside of school at a community event, a park, or home to build rapport.
- The teacher should understand the difference between pressuring the child to talk (e.g., I will reward you if you talk to me) and providing an opportunity and assistance for the child to talk.

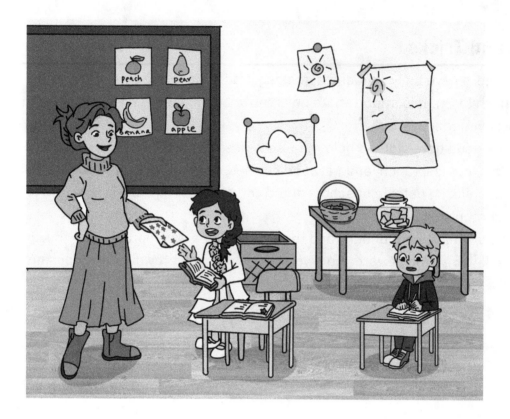

## Communication Book

At the beginning of the school year, to ensure two-way communication between home and school, Amy's homeroom teacher Ms. Lisanne and Amy's parents agreed to communicate daily via a notebook. They assigned Amy the task of passing the communication notebook between Ms. Lisanne and her parents. Ms. Lisanne awarded Amy with a golden star sticker each morning when Amy returned the notebook and jotted down her daily progress, e.g., submitting homework on her own, joining a group activity, raising her hand in maths class, etc.

## Tips and Tricks

- A two-way communication book is very helpful for daily communication, especially when urgent issues need to be addressed promptly, e.g., using the school bathroom. Teachers and parents can communicate about the child's daily needs, concerns, progress, or setbacks. The child is welcome to use the book to communicate with the teacher as well. Parents will reinforce their child's accomplishments at home. In addition to book/email communication, parents can share videos, audio-recordings (e.g., a talking album) with the school to make the child's voice heard.
- Parents and teachers should agree on an action plan and stick to it. They should meet regularly to set goals, formulate action plans, review progress, and make necessary adjustments based on the child's circumstances.
- Identify a supportive adult, a "keyworker" in school. After building a good rapport with the keyworker, the child is willing to talk to and ask for help from them. The communication book can then be phased out.

# The Task Book

The task book aims to help the child initiate a conversation with classmates and all the subject teachers, as well as practise daily communication skills. Parents and the child prepare the task book at home. The tasks are dynamic and change over time with the child's ability and interests. Table 3.2 shows examples of tasks and points of interest, while Form 3.1 shows how the task is tracked in school. The tasks must be within the child's capability and can be revised weekly or monthly. An example of the task can be having an interview/survey for classmates' favourite pets as a journalist or delivering messages as a messenger. Pairing up with a buddy to complete a task together can help reduce anxiety and make it a fun experience. The task book provides the reason for the child to initiate conversation. Once the child completes each task, the teacher or classmate will sign off and/or write a note next to it. If rewards work for your child you may decide to reward your child for carrying these tasks out, in which case a points system could be added.

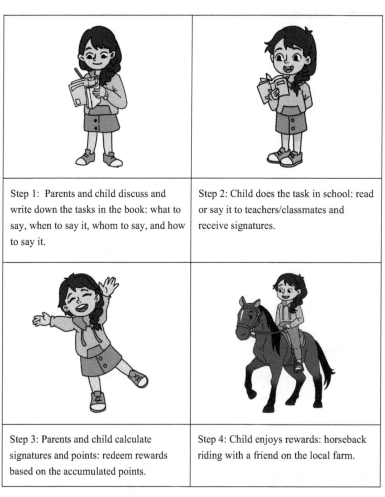

| | |
| --- | --- |
| Step 1: Parents and child discuss and write down the tasks in the book: what to say, when to say it, whom to say, and how to say it. | Step 2: Child does the task in school: read or say it to teachers/classmates and receive signatures. |
| Step 3: Parents and child calculate signatures and points: redeem rewards based on the accumulated points. | Step 4: Child enjoys rewards: horseback riding with a friend on the local farm. |

FIGURE 3.1 How to use the task book

**TABLE 3.2** Tasks and points – Prepare at home and update periodically (this is an example that worked for Amy)

| Tasks | Signature | Calculate Points and Redeem Rewards |
|---|---|---|
| 1 point – Show message or play audio/video recorded at home | 1 point – Classmate | 10 points – Ice cream |
| 2 points – READ or SAY "Here is my homework". "Can I have a pen?" | 2 points – Homeroom teacher | 20 points – Visit the zoo, kayak in the lake |
| 3 points – READ or SAY "Good morning", "Goodbye", and "Thank you" | 3 points – Gym/music teacher | 30 points – Ice-skating, sleepover in a friend's house |
| 4 points – Go with a buddy to do tasks | | 40 points – Picnic in the park |
| | | 50 points – Horseback riding, overnight camping |

# Form 3.1 Tasks Book – Tracking Tasks in School

Teacher/classmates sign on the tasks that child accomplished

| Points | Tasks and associate Points | M | T | W | T | F | Comments |
|---|---|---|---|---|---|---|---|
| 1 | Show message or play audio/video recorded at home | JW AR NX | | | AR | | |
| 2 | READ or SAY "Here is my homework". "Can I have a pen?" | | JW | | | | |
| 3 | READ or SAY "Good morning", "Goodbye", and "Thank you" | | | | | | |
| 4 | Go with a buddy to do tasks | | | | | JW | |

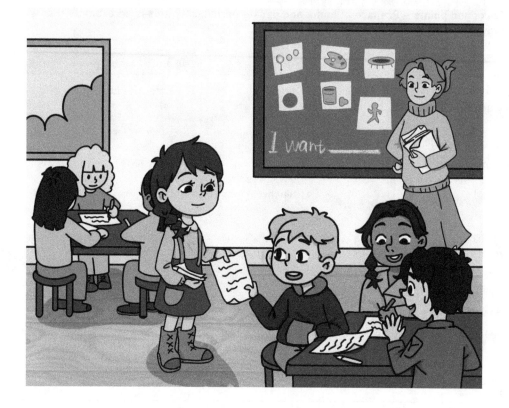

## Language Teacher's Helper and Shadow

As a teacher's helper, Amy had a busy schedule with different tasks assigned by her teacher. She was given the choice of doing it alone or with the help of her talking buddy. Every day, she collected homework from classmates. When Amy found out that no name was written on James's language homework, she managed to communicate with him to add his name by pointing to the blank for NAME, and left the teacher a note with the names of those who did not submit it. Amy checked if the attendance forms were correct before submitting them to the school's main office. She prepared lunch orders using the lunch menu with meal pictures, so her classmates could tell her their orders or point to the pictures. Even though Amy had not talked to most of her classmates yet, she was able to build connections with her peers by doing daily tasks in school, which could also create talking opportunities for her.

## Tips and Tricks

- All children benefit from being given responsibility and feeling valued, and children who have SM are no exception. Ensure they take their turn to assist their teacher.
- Teacher's helper: Assign the child with various tasks throughout the day, such as fixed tasks (e.g., taking daily lunch orders) or spontaneous jobs (e.g., accompanying a classmate to the nurse's office). Allow the child to talk through their talking buddy when needed. It will not only boost the child's confidence but also provide lots of talking opportunities.
- Teacher's shadow: The child is given the opportunity to follow a teacher around for a day and help the teacher with small tasks when asked, e.g., stop by the principal's office to get a letter, go to the garden to water plants, print handouts in the teacher's office, pick up lunch menu from the kitchen, and so on. It makes the child feel special and builds rapport with the teacher.
- By engaging in these appropriate activities/games, the child is under no pressure to speak and feels joyful for participating, which is easier to build rapport between the child and other people.

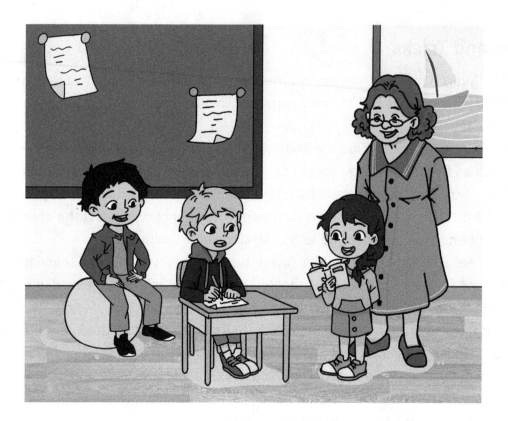

## Language – Support from a Shadow Teacher

Amy had shown significant improvements when her regular teacher spent a few minutes each day or a few times for half an hour each week in school with her, but not all teachers were able to do this. To help accelerate Amy's SM recovery, a shadow teacher was employed by Amy's parents and school to assist Amy in the classroom, as well as in the before and after-school programs.

The shadow teacher, Ms. Rose, had knowledge and experience in SM. She was patient and collaborative. She built rapport with Amy via home visits before seeing Amy in school. Then Ms. Rose served as a "keyworker" to help Amy build confidence, initiate interactions, participate in group/class activities/discussions, and communicate verbally with her peers and teachers. Today, during a group reading activity, Ms. Rose asked Amy to read her favourite story to her talking buddy James and recess buddy, Jeff. She had helped Amy practise reading this story several times. When Jeff and James asked Amy questions about the story, Ms. Rose helped Amy answer by following the 5-second rule and rephrasing the questions as needed.

## Tips and Tricks

- In Amy's case a shadow teacher was used to great advantage. A shadow teacher is normally privately hired by the family of the child with SM. This can help the child build rapport with teachers and classmates. You could ask the school to give a try-out time, e.g, a week/month. When they see the dramatic improvement from the child, they may welcome the shadow teacher to stay longer.

- Hiring a shadow teacher won't be an option available to many people, however this role can be fulfilled by anyone who understands SM and can work in school without disturbing the teaching environment including a child's parent or grandparent. They can assist the child in learning and growing in mainstream classes by providing extra support and attention.

- A shadow teacher keeps open communication between school and parents. It is hard for parents to know exactly what is going on with their child in school. A shadow teacher fills in this gap by being the eyes and ears of the parents, looking out for situations where children are upset or excluded or particularly successful, for example.

- A shadow teacher can help the child academically (e.g., turning in homework assignments), socially (e.g., joining peers in the playground), and communicatively (e.g., asking questions to seek clarification).

- Not every school will be able to incorporate a shadow teacher into their school, but it is a good idea to speak to your setting about options.

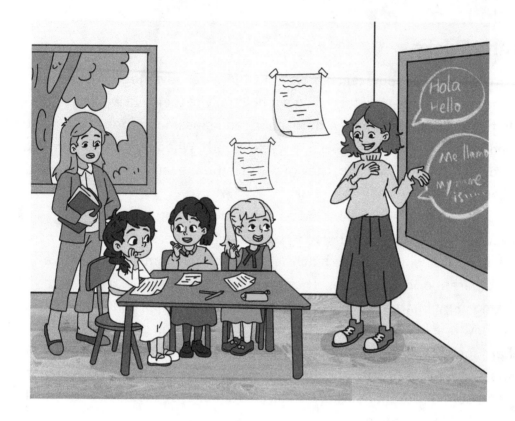

## Private Tutor and School Teacher in After-School Program for Academic and Second Language

Amy's native language was English. As part of the school's academic requirements, Amy chose to study Spanish as a second language. Learning a foreign language was a challenge, especially for Amy. Amy was a perfectionist and did not want to speak until she felt 100% confident. But without practice, Amy's grades fell behind, and she became more and more resistant to the Spanish class.

Seeing Amy's struggle at school, Amy's parents decided to hire a tutor to help her. They found a college student named Catherine, who was playful, soft-spoken, and active. Catherine would accompany Amy to the afterschool program to help Amy with her Spanish assignments, catch up on missed school work, and prepare for the next class. They also played fun games in Spanish at home, which were equivalent to the English version of *Guess Who* or *Hedbanz*. The winner would be rewarded with a treat. They also had regular Spanish lessons a few times a week (30–60 minutes) Catherine helped Amy practise basic language usage, such as Buenos días, gracias, sí, and no, and later moved on to more advanced conversations. They also read in Spanish together and shared the recordings with Amy's Spanish teacher.

## Tips and Tricks

- Attend extracurricular classes to enhance skills, such as English, Math, Language, etc.
- Use voice recordings for desensitisation and play videos of the child speaking English or a second language in a private room with trusted people at school.
- Explore whether the tutor and child can join any after-school program run by one of the child's teachers. The tutor acts as a talking bridge, enabling the child to talk to their teacher outside school. Once the child can talk to their teacher outside school, the conversation can be repeated and continued in school. The teacher can then act as a talking bridge for other children and adults.

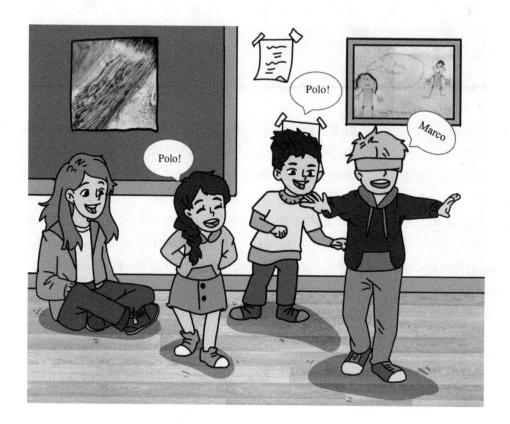

## Academic and After-School Programs, Team Sports, Clubs, and Volunteer Groups

Amy's mom helped Amy try out different after-school programs and sports teams until they found an art class that Amy really enjoyed. Amy could fully immerse herself in the art world without the expectation to speak. A few of Amy's classmates and neighbours were also in the same art class. Amy's big brother Tom came at the end of the class to help Amy play with the other children before it was time to go home. When a classmate with a blindfold called out "Marco", others shouted "Polo" and hid simultaneously. The child would lose if they did not say "Polo" or got caught. Tom shouted "Polo" for Amy at the beginning. Amy realised it was easy to get caught if they were together, so she started to say "Polo" herself and ran in a different direction. The art teacher was happy to stay for a while after class and cheered for them on the side.

Sometimes the teacher would gradually join the game and form a team with Amy to compete with other students. It took little time for the excited Amy to whisper to the teacher about how to win the game.

## Tips and Tricks

- When private or small group playdates are challenging to arrange, look at alternative settings where classmates can meet and join in activities in which the child is interested. School programs are generally better than non-school programs for meeting classmates and transferring progress back to the classroom.

- Suppose the school does not provide sufficient support in school, or parents cannot go to school to help. In that case, these outside school programs allow parents to observe the child's behaviours, coach the teacher, act as a talking bridge, and help to build rapport with classmates/buddies and teachers.

  - After-school programs: Provide an opportunity where children can learn additional skills and meet new schoolmates.
  - Team sports: Active sports that the child enjoys are not only beneficial to a child's physical health but also helpful in boosting their confidence with social interaction. Through their enjoyable competitive sports, children can quickly develop team spirit and build friendships with their teammates.
  - Clubs: Encourage children to meet classmates with common interests/ hobbies.
  - Volunteer groups: Assist children in building self-confidence, gaining self-fulfilment, and developing social skills.

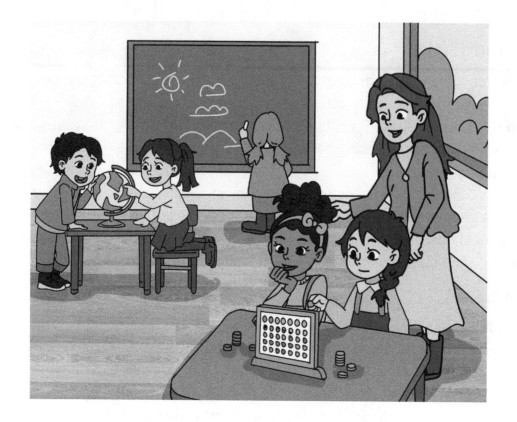

## Maintain Progress during Summer Break

To help Amy stay connected to some of her classmates and teachers, Amy's mom signed Amy up for summer school. Mom requested Amy be placed in the same class as one of her best buddies, Sofie, who was also attending summer school. The two close friends sat at a corner table playing a game. "Amy, what colour do you want, orange or green?" Sofie asked. Amy replied, "green", in a low voice, so others wouldn't hear her. Their teacher, Ms. Jude, came over to check on them every so often. "Looks like you guys are playing a fun game over here". Ms. Jude commented. "Who is winning? Sofie or Amy?" Sofie said, "I think I'm going to". Amy whispered into Sofie's ear, "No, you won't! I'm going to win!" Sofie giggled and repeated to Ms. Jude what Amy had just said.

"Well, I'll have to come back later to see who was right!" said Ms. Jude. "Amy, you don't need to talk to me until you feel ready, okay? I'd like you to talk to Sofie as much as you want. You don't need to keep it a secret".

## Tips and Tricks

- Before the school year ends, parents plan to help the child transition to the next school year. For example, request the child to be placed in a class with a teacher who will be sensitive to the child's struggles. Meet the new teacher before school ends and, if possible, arrange a meeting with the new teacher during summer break outside of school. In addition, request the child's buddies to be placed in the same class to ease the child's transition.

- Find out what the child's classmates are doing during the school break by arranging a summer activity survey. The survey includes the types of activities, who attends, and the location of the activity. The child can choose to attend the same activity with the classmates with whom she/he would like to hang out. By the time school starts, some classmates might have become the child's talking buddies.

- Visit the new school/classroom during summer break and make the second visit right before school begins.

- Summer is an excellent time for the child to meet other children outside school in a more relaxed setting. Use this time to help the child consolidate existing friendships and make new friends. Parents can request a list of new classmates from the school and arrange playdates. Take lots of pictures and videos, and prepare a talking album to share with classmates and teachers after school starts.

- Talk openly about the child's difficulty talking so that they relax and talk freely to their talking buddies, knowing others understand and will not force them to speak.

# Part 4

# CHALLENGES THE CHILD MAY FACE AT SCHOOL

This section focuses on the challenges children with selective mutism (SM) may face in school and provides suggestions for parents and teachers. The child can point to the rooms on the school layout schema to show parents where they have difficulties. Table 4.1 shows a list of activities that the child may encounter both in and outside of school. According to the Anxiety Measurement Hand Chart (Form 1.1, part 1), the child can point to the fingers to help identify their anxiety level for each activity. Parents can use these tools to recognise their children's challenges and strengths.

Furthermore, parents can gain insights into the school challenges from Amy's school life, such as walking into school in the morning, greeting her peers, using the toilet/bathroom, and playing alone during break time/recess. These stories provide practical examples for parents to learn helpful methods and strategies to support their children.

In this section, the authors emphasise the significance of recognising the child's unique talents and skills and providing opportunities for them to showcase these abilities. For instance, the highlight of the butterfly project, subject helpers in technology class, and playing the Chinese harp in music class as potential avenues for showcasing the child's strengths.

The section also highlights the challenges that may arise during holidays, picture day, and in dealing with unhelpful comments and bullies. While some of the solutions may be specific, they have been effective, and parents and teachers are encouraged to find the strategies that work best for their children.

DOI: 10.4324/9781003355267-4

## Identifying Child's Challenge and Providing Support in School

It is quite often that the child cannot express their challenges in school. Let the child identify and mark the room where they feel scared or worried by using a school layout schema. After identifying the challenge, parents and teachers discuss with the child about the possible support. For example, when the child has challenges in music class, instead of singing, let her hand out the instruments to classmates. When the child hesitates to go to the bathroom, pair her with a buddy. When the child is afraid of making mistakes in art class, the teacher lets her sit next to a talking buddy who can help out anytime.

The marks on the school layout schema should be revised periodically. Once the challenge no longer presents itself, mark the room with a smiling face.

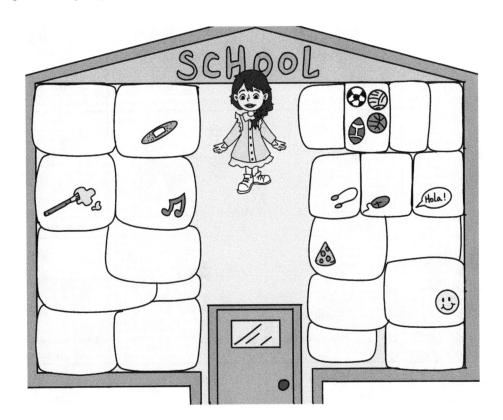

**TABLE 4.1  Talk openly about anxiety and recognise strength/talent/skills**

- Write 1–5 for anxiety level in the box in each situation using the anxiety measurement hand chart and discuss possible solutions.
- Draw a happy face if there is no anxiety issue and recognise strength/talent/skills.

| | | | |
|---|---|---|---|
| ❏ Raise hand and answer questions in classroom | ❏ Present in front of a group of classmates | ❏ Be teacher's helper: Distribute flyers | ❏ Greet teachers and classmates |
| ❏ Play with talking buddy in the playground | ❏ Participate in a small group activity | ❏ Observe and take notes with accompany buddy | ❏ Join Garden club with talking buddy |
| ❏ Paint by oneself | ❏ Paint when teacher is nearby | ❏ Play game with talking buddy | ❏ Play game with buddy when teacher is nearby |
| ❏ Baking playdate with talking buddy at home | ❏ Snow slide playdate | ❏ Horse-riding club | ❏ Animal-petting in school playground |
| ❏ Enter school with teacher | ❏ Shop with aunt | ❏ Camp with parents' friends | ❏ Set up lemonade stand with neighbour |
| ❏ Deliver message and take notes | ❏ Read book to teachers/classmates | ❏ Ask for help from a stranger in a grocery store | ❏ Read to a service dog in a public library |

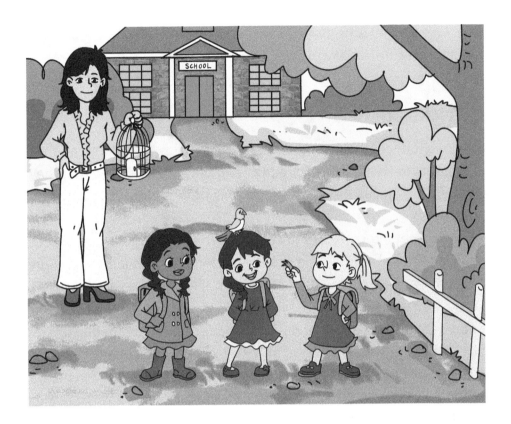

## Meet Classmates/Teachers outside of School in the Morning

Amy had difficulty saying goodbye to her mom before joining others in school each morning. To help Amy tackle this problem, Mom made a few adjustments to the morning routine. They tried arriving at school earlier than other students to get Amy fully warmed up. On their way to school, they would say hello to squirrels busy looking for pine cones and dogs out for morning walks. They would also talk about Amy's daily class schedule, friends and teachers in school, after-school program, upcoming birthday party, and field trip.

Sometimes, Amy would take her parrot Chirp to accompany her to school. Some of Amy's classmates would stop in front of Chirp's cage and say hello. When Chirp said "Squawk!" and "Morning!" Amy and her classmates mimicked happily. When Amy's classmates asked questions regarding Chirp, Mom would act as a "talking bridge" by repeating or rephrasing the questions. Occasionally, Mom would answer the first half of the question and let Amy finish the rest to keep the conversation going.

One morning, Amy put Chirp on her head and prayed so hard that he would not make a mess on her hair. Amy's talking buddies, Sofie and Isabella, greeted Amy and Chirp enthusiastically. Like magic, Amy gave Chirp back to Mom and said goodbye, then walked into school hand-in-hand with Sofie and Isabella.

## Tips and Tricks

- SM child takes longer to warm up due to their sensitivity. Be patient and respect their pace. Parents can help the child prepare/visualise their day the night before. Discuss the child's concerns, offer solutions and give reassurance.
- Pets can be a great intermediary to connect the child to their peers. The child can also use a stuffed animal or a voice-recording toy instead of a real pet. The child can practise making animal sounds, such as "Sssss", "Zzzzz", or "Roar" before saying words.
- Parent stays at the child's side and helps by offering talking opportunities until the child can speak to a potential friend. Use graded questions (page 76) to ease the child into speaking to the parent in front of the new friend. Parent acts as a go-between, relaying requests and questions between the children until, eventually, the child talks directly to the new friend.

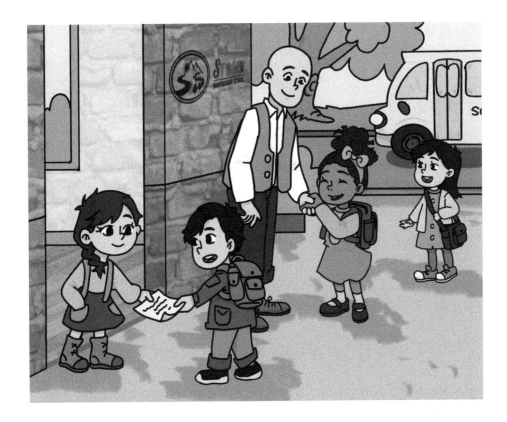

## Greet Teachers and Students

Mr. Alex was Amy's counsellor and noticed Amy never said "hi" or "good morning" when she entered school in the morning. To help Amy warm up in the morning and greet, Mr. Alex asked Amy to be the greeting student, standing next to him in the morning.

Amy, and sometimes Amy's buddy would arrive at school 15 minutes earlier before the school gate opened. Mr. Alex then would do a warm-up session with them. They would play games, watch Amy and her friends' playdate videos, and start conversations in Mr. Alex's office. Afterwards, Amy went with Mr. Alex to greet students at the front gate. As Mr. Alex greeted each student, Amy stood next to Mr. Alex and tried to memorise everyone's name. Amy could also choose to press the button on her stuffed animal to deliver a recorded voice message, such as "Good morning!" or "Happy Birthday!"

Sometimes, Mr. Alex would ask Amy to help distribute school trip flyers, give out birthday gifts, and say "Happy Birthday" if the birthday child happened to be her buddy. In the beginning, Amy greeted together with Mr. Alex or played her recorded message, and sometimes they said "hi" in a loud, silly, and funny animal voice when

Amy's talking buddy passed by. Over time, Amy was able to say "hi" to most of the students and teachers with a big smile on her face.

## Tips and Tricks

- Teachers should greet children with a smile and understand that the child is not being rude if they don't answer back. Reassure the child that non-verbal replies (wave or smile) are acceptable.
- Rehearse greetings with the teacher and talking buddies when no one is around.

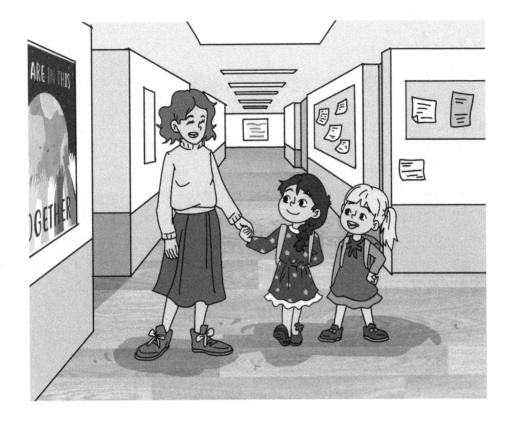

## Walk to the Building with Classmates/Teacher in the Morning

Amy seemed relaxed and was able to communicate verbally when she arrived outside of school in the morning. However, she stopped talking after entering the school's front gate. Therefore, Ms. Cookie tried to meet Amy and her talking buddy Sofie in front of the school in the morning. They chatted about Amy's pet bird, Chirp, Ms. Cookie's dog Marley, and Sofie's upcoming birthday party. Seeing Amy enjoying these topics, Ms. Cookie walked them into school and kept the conversations going.

Since it was still early and nobody else was around, Amy continued to talk.

When they reached the classroom where Amy felt most anxious, Ms. Cookie immediately assigned Amy as the teacher's helper for the day. Amy would help Ms. Cookie set up the classroom, distribute worksheets, prepare lunch orders, etc. "Ms. Cookie, is Jeff coming today? I didn't see his lunch order". Amy asked. "He is out for today". Ms. Cookie replied. "Ms. Cookie, there aren't enough worksheets". Amy counted the worksheet and asked. "Please go with Sofie to the front office to get extra copies." Ms. Cookie responded. "Amy, you ask for copies, and Sofie, please help Amy if she needs help", Ms. Cookie added.

## Tips and Tricks

- Children rise to a challenge more easily when they know there is a back-up plan.
- Catch the talking momentum and prolong it by keeping the child busy with tasks they are capable of and interested in doing. Pair them up with a talking buddy to reduce anxiety and provide support.
- When assigning tasks, the teacher ensures that the child knows exactly what to do or say. It may require rehearsal through role-play in advance.
- Gradually help the child initiate verbal or non-verbal interactions by letting them do as much as possible on their own, playing games where they ask questions, give clues, and issue instructions, and by losing the habit of prompting the child in turn-taking activities.

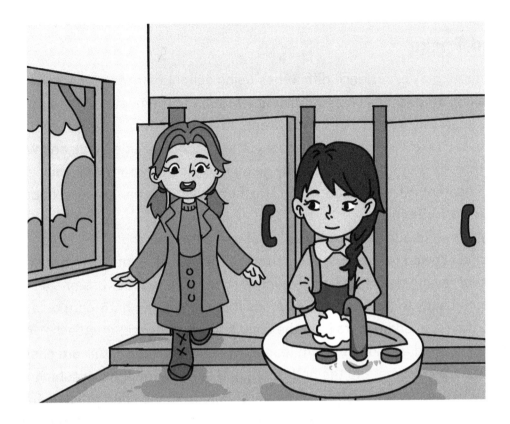

## Go to the Bathroom with a Bathroom Buddy

Amy's teacher, Ms. Lisanne, reminded Amy and her assigned bathroom buddy to use the bathroom every hour to avoid accidents. Today Ms. Lisanne asked, "Amy, would you please go to the bathroom with our new classmate, Marissa, and show her the cafeteria and water fountain on the way back?" That was a magical turning point. Amy had been the one accepting help in the past, but today she could help others. On their way to the bathroom, Amy and Marissa were able to talk about the school, classes, and social events. "Do you like this school?" Marissa asked. "Kind of, but it's also kind of..." Amy responded. A simple bathroom trip turned into a break-the-ice activity!

## Tips and Tricks

- SM children may experience difficulties using school bathrooms because they fear asking for permission and drawing attention to themselves. Therefore, it is a top priority for teachers and parents to address this issue early on. Parents can take their child to practise before school, after school, and when the bathroom is unoccupied. Start by going into the bathroom with your child, then the parent retreats to outside or further away. Practising with a buddy may be more effective.

- To help the child alleviate the pressure of using the bathroom, the child should be allowed to use a sign to notify the teacher of a bathroom break instead of raising their hand and asking verbally. The teacher assigns a bathroom buddy to the child and reminds them to use the bathroom on a regular basis. In addition, to help the child build confidence, the teacher can appoint the child as the bathroom leader, who can give out bathroom passes, accompany a classmate to the bathroom, and enforce the hand-washing rule.

- Parents/teacher/child's bathroom buddy should help the child practise using the bathroom not only at home and school but also at other places, such as in a restaurant, at a mall, or at a friend's house.

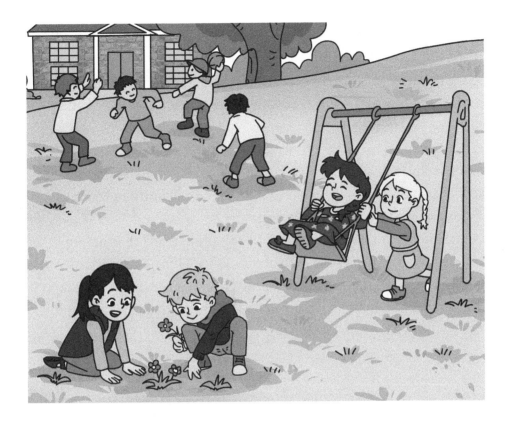

## School Challenge – Break Time/Recess

During recess, among all the children running, playing, and laughing, it was hard not to notice a girl who stood on the side silently. Amy wanted to join others, but she did not know how. She usually played by herself or just watched everyone else play. Amy's homeroom teacher and Amy's parents worked together to build a buddy system to help Amy with different challenges in school.

Amy's recess buddy Sam came over and suggested to Amy, "Let's go to the swing set". A smile appeared on Amy's face. "Amy, let me push you first. Just call out 'stop' when it is too high for you!" The swing got higher and higher, becoming too high for Amy. "Stop", Amy called out to Sam, but no one could hear her. After trying a few times, Amy had to yell out, "Stop!" It was loud and clear, and everyone heard it. "You had one of the highest swings I have ever seen", said Ms. Lana, who had been watching Amy for a long time. Amy pointed at Sam with a smile and said, "Because she could not hear me!" Sam and Amy then walked hand-in-hand toward the flower-picking group.

## Tips and Tricks

- Activities with verbal/non-verbal communication, body movement, teamwork, competition, and fun/exciting play are the best to promote the child's vocalisation.

- Start communication in a one-on-one situation. Once the child communicates with a buddy in a "safe area" where no one pays attention, expand this approach to a small group activity. Help the child to continue talking while returning to the classroom from recess.

- In gym class, either indoor or outdoor, the child may be too tense to move freely, thus unable to follow the instruction to run, jump, act or join the group activities. To create opportunities to participate, the teacher can assign the child and her/his buddy or small group to the same or easier activities at the side or some distance from the big crowd.

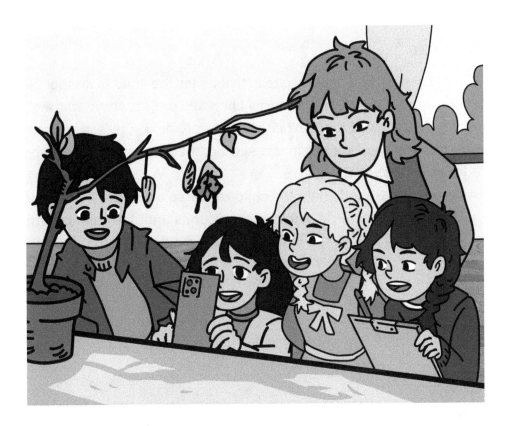

## Butterfly Project 1 – Classroom Observation

Ever since Amy visited a butterfly house at the botanical garden with her parents, she became fascinated with the life cycle of butterflies. She even asked her parents to purchase *"A Butterfly's Life Cycle"* book to learn more about it. At last, she got some butterfly chrysalises to have more hands-on experience.

Amy brought the chrysalis cage to show to her friends at the garden club in school. The club's instructor, Ms. Bo, assigned Amy and three of her friends to observe and track the butterfly's life changes. The children put down their observations on a chart, along with their drawing illustrations. Amy and her "butterfly buddies" were also responsible for cleaning up the cage and watering the plant. Ms. Bo also asked the butterfly team to record videos explaining each stage in a butterfly's life. Since Amy had learned so much from reading the butterfly book, she volunteered to be the narrator in the videos. "A caterpillar is inside the pupa. Its body changes over the next two weeks". Amy memorised her lines from the butterfly book. These videos were recorded at home and later shared with Mr. Alex and Amy's classmates.

## Tips and Tricks

- Parents and teachers find appropriate activities for the child to create more talking opportunities. The butterfly chrysalis project above was a great activity that allowed the teacher and peers to hear Amy's voice for the first time. Once Amy had spoken in one setting, the same activity could be repeated in other settings.
- Parents or supportive adults help the child rehearse activities/situations/ conversations in advance. Practise for a few rounds until the child is familiar with the sequence of events and language used in different situations.

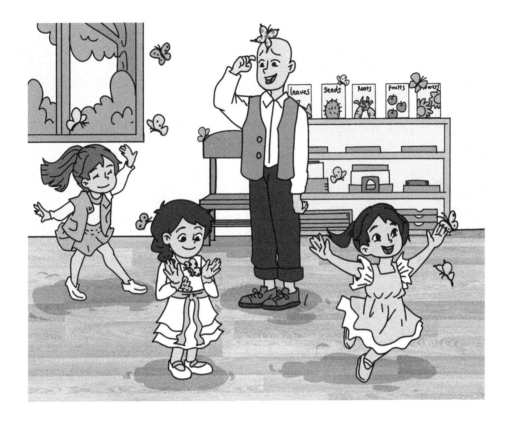

## Butterfly Project 2 – Bring Butterflies to School Counsellor's Office

Amy brought her butterfly cage to Mr. Alex's office for their weekly meeting.

Amy had never spoken to Mr. Alex before but enjoyed her time with him. Amy's butterfly buddy, Sabrina, joined them too. First, they watched the butterfly videos narrated by Amy. Then Amy and Sabrina took turns reading *"A Butterfly's Life Cycle"* book to Mr. Alex. "A female monarch butterfly floats in the air...". Amy began reading in a low voice. Her voice got louder and more confident after a few rounds. After that, they did a butterfly quiz and finished with butterfly crafts.

Finally, the big day was here. After two weeks of waiting, butterflies broke out from chrysalises. Amy invited her "butterfly buddies" to Mr. Alex's office to release the butterflies from the cage. The children were so excited to see beautiful butterflies flying around and chasing after them. Everyone laughed when a butterfly landed on Mr. Alex's head. Children took turns counting the number of butterflies and naming different colour variations. Amy had been comfortably talking during this entire process. No one commented on it since everyone was preoccupied with butterflies.

## Tips and Tricks

- Voice/video recordings are an effective way to help the child desensitise. Allowing their voice to be heard by others with no adverse consequences is a significant milestone in overcoming SM. Parents can make a habit of recording their child's daily activities so that it is not unusual for the child to share videos with family members and hear their own voices. Sharing these recordings with teachers is then a more routine activity.

- After building rapport with the child, the supportive adult can read together with the child their favourite books or passages. Parents can help the child practise reading ahead of time before reading aloud to the adult.

- Taking all pressure off children to talk can result in good rapport but won't necessarily lead to talking. Notice that a few minutes of one-on-one talking with the teacher every day is better than a half hour weekly session. Reading and rehearsed lines are much easier for SM children than conversation, so create a need to speak using these earlier stages of communication.

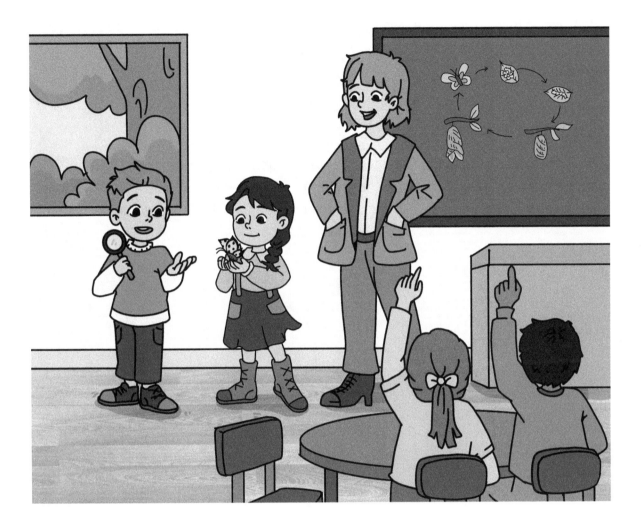

## Butterfly Project 3 – Show and Tell

Amy and her parents agreed to use the butterfly for Show and Tell in school this week as part of her task and reward plan. Amy had learned so much about butterflies from reading books and observing chrysalis. She was eager to share her learnings with her classmates. Amy first wrote down what she would say for her Show and Tell. Then, her parents helped her rehearse her speech several times at home. Amy also rehearsed with her teacher during the one-on-one time and in a small group with a few talking buddies. To help Amy feel less anxious, she was paired up with her talking buddy, Noah, to do the Show and Tell together. Both Amy's parents and teacher reassured Amy that if she did not want to talk, she could show while Noah could tell.

When it was Show and Tell time, Amy got a little nervous, but rehearsals and having Noah beside her helped a lot. In the beginning, Amy played a video of her explaining the butterfly life cycle. Then she showed the butterfly to the class and read from her notes. When it was Q&A time, she answered some questions she had rehearsed at home. Noah helped her with other questions that were a little too difficult for her to answer.

## Tips and Tricks

- Rehearsals at home or in school before the actual presentation really help.
- Prepare an escape route for the child to feel less anxious.
- Assign a buddy to support the child in completing a challenging task.

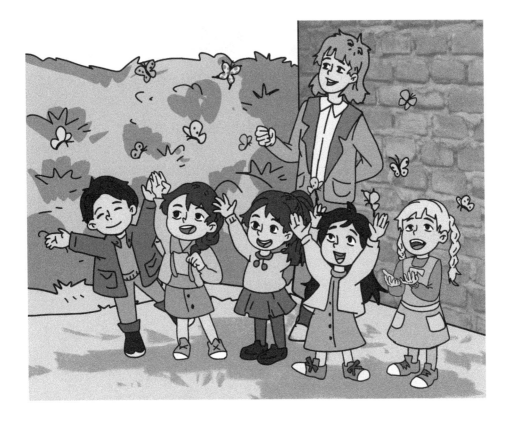

## Butterfly Project 4 – Release Butterflies into Nature

After the butterflies came out of the chrysalises, the garden club students observed them closely for a few days. The butterflies were let out of the cage and flying in the classroom. They landed on children's shoulders, arms, hands, and hair. One butterfly landed on Amy's homework. "This butterfly wants to do my homework!" Amy giggled. Then this butterfly flew around the classroom and stopped at each child's table. Amy joked, "This is a social butterfly". Everyone laughed and agreed with her. Ms. Bo observed the children on the side. She was pleased to see Amy make so much progress over the past few weeks.

It was time to release the butterflies into nature. Amy and her classmates planned the release in the school garden on a sunny afternoon. When the "social butterfly" flew away, Amy called out, "Bye, Yellow, go and find your new home!" Children took turns waving and saying goodbye to the butterflies, "Bye-bye, Red!" "Bye, Blue. I will miss you". Ms. Bo took a video to capture this wonderful moment.

## Tips and Tricks

- Bring an interesting project or activity the child enjoys doing at home to school.
- Activities involved with animals and insects can help open up the communication channel between the child and teachers/classmates. It is easier to talk to animals as they don't ask questions like people do! Animals have a way of capturing our attention and making us laugh. Teaching puppy tricks is a lovely way to practise simple commands with friends.
- Help the child stand out and be the project leader to build their confidence in speaking.

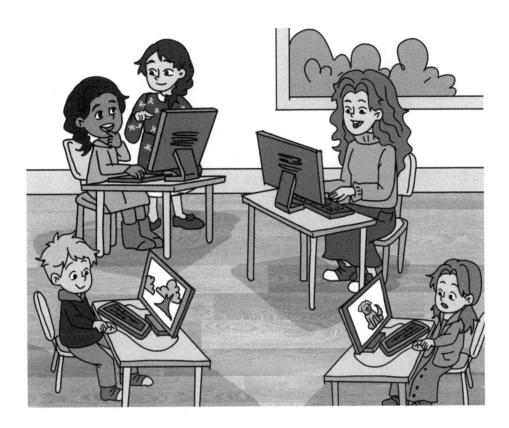

## Subject Helper in Technology Class

Amy faced challenges in all subjects as long as they related to communication. In technology class, she was afraid to communicate about her computer issues, such as a broken mouse, and what to do after she finished her work. Because Amy was good at computer graphics, the subject teacher, Ms. Carole, asked Amy to be her helper since Amy always finished her work quickly and correctly. Today in class, Amy was the first to finish her work. After checking Amy's work, Ms. Carole announced, "Amy has finished her work. If anyone needs help, please either come to me or Amy".

"Amy, come here!" talking buddy Isabella said, "I'm drawing a little girl now, but her hair is crooked". Amy demonstrated and explained how to straighten the hair. Then Marissa called out, "Amy, my computer is down". Amy thought... I'm only six years old, and I can't fix your computer. So, she walked up to Ms. Carole for help. Amy patted lightly on Ms. Carole's shoulder and whispered, "Marissa's computer is down". Ms. Carole then went to help Marissa. "Amy, come and see the tree I drew. It's too small for me to draw a squirrel on it". "Amy, how come my kitten looks like a puppy?" Other students were calling out to Amy for help. Amy felt busy but proud.

## Tips and Tricks

- Find a subject the child is interested in or good at and ask to be the subject helper. Being a subject helper not only helps with a child's confidence and keeps them busy but also increases their interactions with their peers and the subject teacher.
- Parents can ask to communicate with the subject teacher in advance to help the child preview the content of the next class. This way, the child can complete classwork more quickly and correctly, leaving time to help their peers.

# Form 4.1 Teacher's Helper/Subject Helper Work Tracking

1. Being a teacher's helper will create talking opportunities, increase self-confidence, and build rapport with classmates and teachers.
2. Work examples: Collect/distribute homework, place lunch orders, organise bookshelf, deliver notes, sharpen pencils, accompany a classmate to the bathroom/front office/nurse's office, clean tables, mop the floor, etc. Work can be completed with/without verbal communication.
3. EACH subject teachers add name, month, date, work, and initials in the cell for the day.
4. This can also serve as a weekly communication sheet between parents and teachers.

| Teacher: | | Month | | From _____ | | To_____ |
|---|---|---|---|---|---|---|
| | Work | Monday | Tuesday | Wednesday | Thursday | Friday |
| 1 | | | | | | |
| 2 | | | | | | |
| 3 | | | | | | |
| 4 | | | | | | |
| 5 | | | | | | |

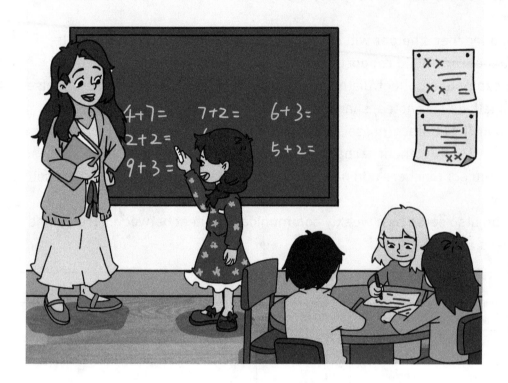

## Answer Questions in Class with Support

It happened quite often that Amy raised her hand when the teacher asked questions, but she was unable to answer. Nevertheless, Amy's teacher Ms. Pear would still call on Amy to give her an opportunity to speak. Ms. Pear waited for 5 seconds for Amy to respond, and then, if there was no answer, she rephrased the question so that Amy could nod or shake her head, tell her talking buddy the answer, or write her answer on the board.

Ms. Pear also allowed Amy to pre-record her answer to present in class and paired Amy with her talking buddy to do presentations together. The more Amy's voice was heard in class, the easier it became for her to answer Ms. Pear when she put her hand up.

## Tips and Tricks

- Show empathy: The teacher tells the child that he/she understands how difficult it is for the child to speak and other people out there have similar experiences. The teacher reassures the child that it is just a matter of time before they can talk to anyone.
- Show Support: The teacher includes the child in all verbal/non-verbal activities and assists them with talking opportunities regardless of the outcomes. The teacher accepts all forms of communication from the child, whether it is written, pre-recorded, gestures, or via the child's talking buddies.
- Observe the child's behaviour, identify the child's communication stage, facilitate and prompt conversation to the next stage by asking graded questions and accept all forms of communication. For example, when the child is in stage one, the teacher can ask the child to communicate by writing, nodding, and pointing. The teacher should use strategies to help children nudge their communication to the next stage till children can comfortably speak whenever needed.
- Share the child's SM information with school staff and other adults, so they can support the child whenever and with whatever they need. Everyone in the child's school life who knows the child is encouraged to learn about SM and how to interact with the child.

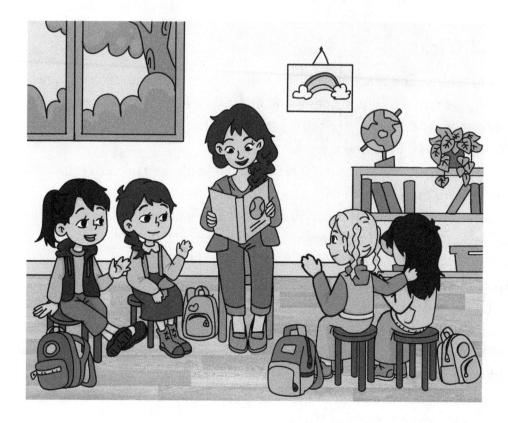

## Read and Discussion Time in the Library

In the school's library, Amy, her talking buddy Sam, and two other classmates were sitting around Ms. Lena, the librarian. "Today, we will take turns reading a book about animals together". Ms. Lena showed the book to everyone and started reading the first sentence. Before this reading session, Amy had been able to read in front of Ms. Lena and Sam. But it was too much to read in front of the whole class. When it was Amy's turn, it took her 5 seconds to get ready and read her part.

More turns went by, Amy's voice became more audible, and now everyone could hear her. Then it was discussion time. Ms. Lena asked, "Who can tell me which animal was smarter in the story?" All the kids raised their hands, including Amy. Ms. Lena picked Amy to give her a chance to speak. Amy smiled and said, "Fox!"

## Tips and Tricks

- Provide the child with an opportunity to answer a question if they raise their hand. During the class discussion, give hints/help for possible answers, and accept both verbal and non-verbal responses, such as nodding, pointing, or writing. The child can also choose to answer through their talking buddy; it may be very quiet at first but will get louder.

- Adhere to the 5-second rule. When asking a question, wait five seconds for the child to think and prepare their answer. If there is no answer after 5 seconds, the teacher can rephrase the question or lower the difficulty of answering (graded questions), so that the child can answer by nodding or shaking their head or pointing. For example, if Amy had not said "Fox", Ms. Lena could have passed her the book and asked her to point to the smartest animal.

- If there is still no answer, the teacher can ask the child to talk through their talking buddy, or simply comment "I can see you are thinking hard about that," and moves on.

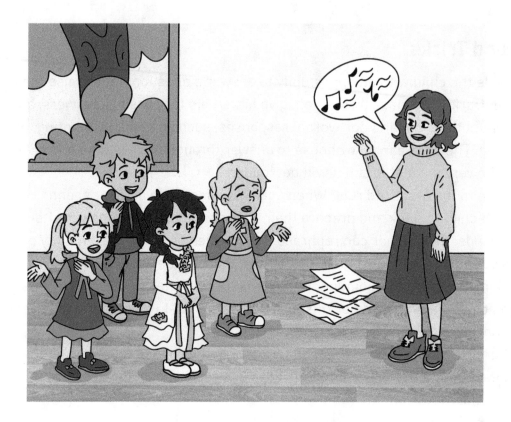

## Music Class

Amy enjoyed music, and she had been playing Guzheng, a Chinese Harp, for two years. Despite all her efforts, Amy could not overcome her fear of being heard by others. She stood quietly when Ms. Cookie, the music teacher, instructed the class to sing together. "I know this song! I can sing it at home". Amy thought to herself. She tried to move her lips, but nothing came out.

Ms. Cookie later learned about Amy's unique situation and was more than willing to help by making a few changes/exceptions in her class. Firstly, she moved Amy from being in the front of the class to the back corner so that Amy would not feel like the centre of attention and thus alleviate her stress. Secondly, Ms. Cookie invited Amy to participate in the class non-verbally, e.g., by holding the music notes, monitoring the music record, or flipping the Powerpoint presentation on the computer. Instead of singing, Amy could choose to play an instrument for her peers to dance to. She could also pre-record her singing or dancing at home and show the video to the class. These videos would let Amy's classmates get to know her and show what she could do and how beautiful her voice could be. Lastly, Ms. Cookie asked Amy to be her assistant, pass out instruments, collect musical notes, or return the instruments to the shelves.

## Tips and Tricks

- The teacher should be informed that a child with SM is in their class and be equipped with basic SM knowledge to help the child. For example, the teacher knows not to pressure the child to speak, sing, or dance, yet finds other ways to include the child in class participation.
- The teacher accepts alternative methods of communication and assigns the child with manageable tasks to build confidence and create talking opportunities. Build a safety net for the child by seating him/her strategically towards the back of the room and surrounded by his/her buddies.
- Tell the child you understand that talking is difficult at the moment, but singing is different from talking. Singing won't lead to lots of questions or conversations, so it's safe for the child to try if they feel like it.

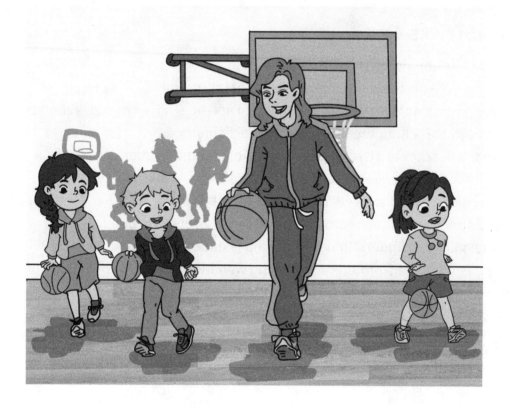

## Practice Physical Activities in a Small Group before Doing It with Whole Class

Physical activities were not Amy's strong suit. She was afraid her classmates would laugh at her if she appeared to be clumsy in her PE class. As such, she chose to stand on the side and watch others playing instead. After meeting with Amy's parents about Amy's condition and the reasons behind her opt-out, Mr. Bill invited Amy for a private tour of the school gym. He briefly introduced the PE class routine and activities, then showed her different sports equipment. Mr. Bill assured Amy that she wouldn't be picked out to do a demonstration unless she volunteered. He also told Amy that it was okay to ask questions through her talking buddy if she was unsure what to do. She could also use non-verbal communication, like nodding and pointing, until she became comfortable using words with him.

The following day, Mr. Bill invited Amy and her talking buddies for a small group tour. During the tour, the children were excited to try out different equipment. Mr. Bill demonstrated how to dribble a basketball and make a 3-pointer. Children were eager to try out and were given basketballs to practise. Amy had been practising basketball at home, as recommended by Mr. Bill to Amy's parents. Amy dribbled the ball and passed it around to her buddies. Everyone had a fantastic time and workout.

## Tips and Tricks

- Parents and teachers should work together to help the child participate in physical activities. Do not let SM impact a child's health and physical development.
- Teachers should encourage the child's participation, track the child's progress, and offer praise when the child tries out something new. "Amy, you did a good job of controlling the ball," "Wow, you can run really fast!" "Amy, good job by passing the ball to your teammate..."

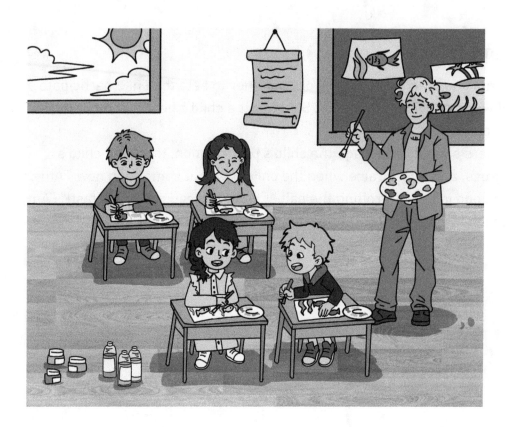

## Ask for Help in Art Class

Amy liked to paint, and she painted very well. Her drawing was displayed in the local library and art gallery. She felt very relaxed and at ease during the painting lessons. She could focus on drawing instead of worrying about speaking and answering questions as in other classes.

The painting teacher, Mr. Bobby, announced to the students: "Today, we are going to do a watercolour painting of the ocean. Please use your imagination and paint what you think the ocean should look like and what ocean animals live there". Mr. Bobby looked at Amy and continued, "Amy, can you please help distribute the drawing paper, brush, and watercolour paints to everyone (assign Amy as a teacher's helper). Amy got up and did what Mr. Bobby asked her to do.

Amy stopped in the middle of her painting because she ran out of green paint. She was debating what to do. Luckily, Amy's talking buddy James was sitting next to her. James noticed something was bothering Amy and asked, "Amy, is there anything wrong?" Amy replied in a low voice, "I need more green paint". "I can go with you to ask Mr. Bobby for it". James gladly offered his help. They went together to see Mr. Bobby. Mr. Bobby smiled and asked, "How can I help?" After a few seconds of pause, Amy asked Mr. Bobby, "Can I have the green paint?"

## Tips and Tricks

- Sit the child with their buddies to get timely support. This also helps reduce the child's anxiety when they encounter a problem.
- Parents help enhance the child's art skills at home so that the child can feel more confident to draw/paint in class.

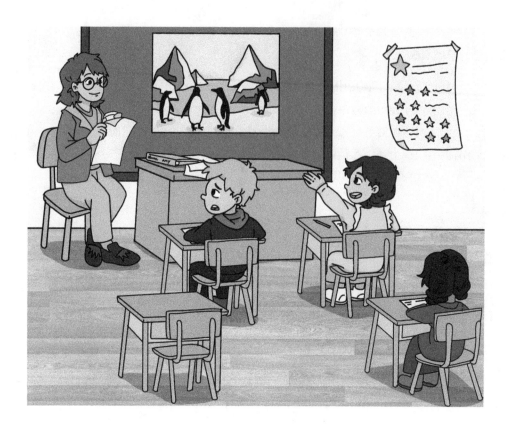

## Science Substitute Teacher

"Hi, I'm Ms. Andy, your substitute teacher for today. I'll be teaching science. Good morning, everyone!" "Good morning, Ms. Andy!" Amy greeted Ms. Andy along with her classmates. "Okay, let's start with attendance". When Ms. Andy called out names, classmates shouted, "Here!" When Amy was called, she waved at the teacher.

Ms. Andy asked, "Can anyone tell me where penguins live?" Amy slowly raised her hand while other classmates were still thinking of the answer. "Amy, what's your answer?" Amy looked at Ms. Andy and hesitated. Ms. Andy then asked the question in a different way: "Do penguins live at the South Pole or the North Pole?" Amy still didn't answer. After waiting for another five seconds, Ms. Andy walked to Amy, smiled, and said quietly, "North" (pointing up), "or South"(pointing down). Amy pointed down straightaway. "Excellent, Amy", said Ms. Andy, "That's exactly right". Amy beamed.

Ms. Andy continued asking questions while slowly returning to her desk. "Is Antarctica cold or hot?... Do you know any other animals that live in Antarctica?" When Amy put her hand up again, Ms. Andy moved over to her, and this time, Amy was able to answer. Gradually Ms. Andy pulled back, and Amy had to raise her voice so that Ms. Andy could hear her. By the end of the lesson, Amy was able to answer questions in her normal voice.

## Tips and Tricks

- Parents and teachers can create a folder on how to communicate with the SM child, e.g., allowing the child to wave instead of saying "here" when doing roll-call.
- Teacher informs parents in advance about the substitute teacher and the lesson content, so the child knows what to expect.
- Parents and teachers can use the home-school communication book to update the child's daily needs and progress.

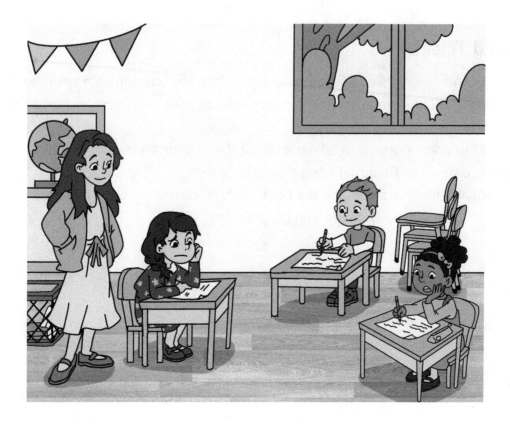

## Take a Test

Amy dreaded taking exams, especially today's test when she realised she had forgotten to bring a pencil. Amy was too afraid to speak up and ask for help. So she sat there and stared at the blank paper. Amy's teacher finally noticed her and went to check if she needed help. After getting a pencil from the teacher, Amy was able to complete the first page of her exam. However, since she lost too much time in the beginning, she could not complete the remainder of her exam. "I knew it. My grades will never be good". Amy thought to herself, feeling down.

Amy was a bright girl and should be able to take tests. However, her grades did not reflect her academic abilities and were on the lower end of the curve. Several factors impacted her grades. Amy missed turning in some of her assignments, fearing that she would have to present in front of the class. It took her longer to get warmed up to unfamiliar subject teachers, thus delaying her learning progress. Her worry about going to the bathroom distracted her from studying in class. On top of that, she was too afraid to seek clarification from teachers when she did not understand. Some SM children may exhibit a perfectionist personality trait. While they may excel on the initial section of a test and score full marks, their perfectionism may cause them to run out of time before completing the rest of the questions.

## Note

1 Johnson, M. & Wintgens, A. (2016). The selective mutism resource manual, 2ed, Speechmark Publishing.

## Tips and Tricks

- A child with SM often goes unnoticed because of their quiet nature. If the teacher is too busy to monitor the child closely, they can assign a few students to be the child's buddies for periodic check-ups, e.g., "Do you need anything? What is wrong? Why did you stop writing?"
- If speaking is too challenging at that moment at school, the child can practise expressing their needs at home. Following a discussion with the teacher, the parent can help the child to find and act out ways to express themselves non-verbally whenever they need help. For example, pointing to flashcards/pictures, writing down their requests, pre-recording their needs on a recording device, etc.
- Some children do not submit work assignments because they are afraid of being called on to read their good work. Ask teachers to reassure the children that this will not happen unless they volunteer.
- Tests can take various forms, such as oral (e.g., singing, reading, reciting, presenting), written on paper, computer-based, performance-based (e.g., on stage), or physical (e.g., running in the gym). Each type of test presents different challenges for the child. It can be discouraging if a child knows the subject well but receives a low grade due to test anxiety. In such cases, teachers and parents should prepare and offer alternative methods to accommodate the child's needs during exams.[1]

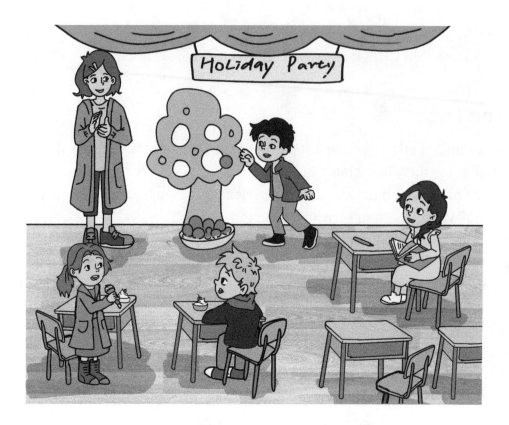

## Holiday Party

Hooray! The holiday party prepared by students and several volunteer parents was about to begin. The usually quiet classroom was now filled with cheerful laughter. The grand "Holiday Party" banner was hanging on the wall. The students were playing different games around the classroom. Jeff was throwing balls to go through an apple tree made of cardboard. Ms. Kerri was cheering for him on the side. Everyone laughed when the ball missed the hole and bounced back, hitting Jeff's head. James was listening to Marissa singing. "Wow, she really has a good voice". Amy thought to herself. Classmates were chatting and giggling. The room was filled with a festive atmosphere.

There was, however, one person who was not celebrating on this special occasion. It was Amy. She sat quietly behind her desk, watching Jeff play. Amy wanted to participate, but surrounded by so many unfamiliar parents and classmates, "I'd better stay put... unless someone calls me", Amy said to herself.

As if Amy's wish was heard, Cate ran over and said, "Hey, Amy, the teacher asked us to help her distribute the cake". Cate took Amy's hand and dragged her towards the cake table. "Come on, let's do it together". Amy nodded. "Chocolate cake?" Amy handed the plate to David. "Can you get me one too? I want vanilla, thank you", said Sofie, who was playing chess with David. "Okay, one moment", Amy responded with a smile. Amy distributed snacks and drinks, helped collect trash, and walked around the classroom among the activity groups to see who needed help. She was busy and had no time for rest. Yet she was so happy because helping others was her favourite thing.

"Amy, come to play the apple tree game", Jeff shouted across the classroom. "Coming", Amy shouted back without realising how loud she was. Ms. Kerri praised Amy at the end of the party for her excellent participation. Amy had a fantastic time.

## Tips and Tricks

- Parents can offer to be a volunteer at a holiday party to help the child feel more supported. Tell the child in advance about the time, location, who will attend, and what will happen at the party.
- It is challenging for the child to take the initiative to participate. Assign a buddy to invite the child to class activities/games/conversations.
- Keep the child busy by assigning small tasks to them. The child will not only feel accomplished but also less anxious in a crowded and noisy environment.

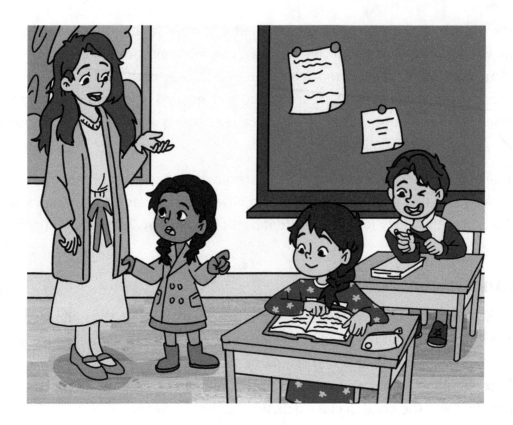

## Watch Out for Unhelpful Comments and Bullies

One day in class, Amy's classmate Isabella asked Ms. Pear, "Why does Amy never talk to us? Can she talk at all?" Ms. Pear replied, "Yes, Amy can talk. She talks to her family at home. She is just not ready to talk in school yet". "Amy needs our help to bring her voice into school. When she finally talks in school, let's not act surprised because she has always been able to talk". Ms. Pear went on, "Would you like to be her recess buddy?" Isabella nodded with a big smile, "Sure, I'd love to". Other classmates were eager to help and volunteered to be Amy's lunch buddy, bathroom buddy, gym buddy, and so on.

## Tips and Tricks

- Talk to the child about reactions from other people: SM children worry about other people's reactions when they hear his/her voice. Parents and teachers should discuss with the child about their fear and concerns in order to take the next step forward.
- Involve the child's classmates: Depending on the child's age group, teachers can talk openly to the class about the child's SM and ask for their support (when the child is not present). Parents or teachers may also consider sending SM information sheets to other classmates' parents in order to get united support in the classroom. It will also serve as a stepping stone to a playdate invitation.
- Teachers, parents, and the child should come up with a non-verbal way to communicate in case of emergency or a safe haven to retreat to, such as pointing to the pictures to express his/her needs.
- Not all inappropriate behaviours are considered bullying at a young age. Young children are still developing proper social skills and etiquette. However, it is important to consider that a child with SM may easily be targeted because they are unable to tell an authority figure if anyone says or does something to upset them. Teachers and buddies should be aware of this and keep an eye out for any rising issues.

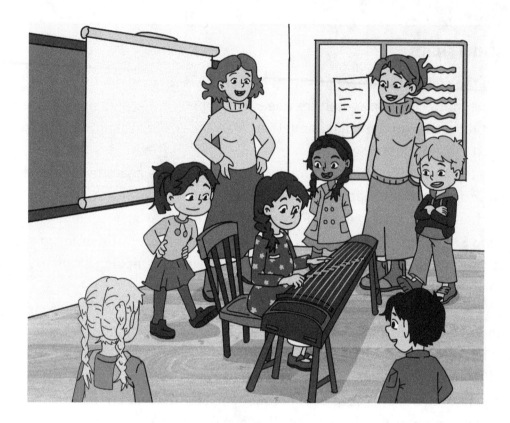

## Showcase Talent/Skills – Essential Component No. 7 in the Recovery Journey – Chinese Harp (Guzheng) Performance in the Music Class

One effective way to support a child's growth and development is to identify their unique talents and interests, help them develop the skills, and create opportunities for them to showcase their abilities and participate in activities.

The school talent show was coming up. Amy's mom encouraged Amy to showcase her Guzheng, an ancient Chinese musical instrument that Amy had played for two years, but Amy was reluctant to take part. Mom assured Amy that she would also play Guzheng in the back in case of any mistake on stage. Mom walked Amy through everything that Amy needed to know for the talent show: her spot on the stage, how to get on and off the stage, how many people would be attending, and how the audience would react before and after her performance.

To help Amy rehearse her musical piece and get used to being the centre of attention, Amy's music teacher, Ms. Cookie, invited Amy to perform in a music class before going onto the big stage. However, before that, she paired Amy with Amy's talking buddy Cate to announce the performance and chant a Chinese poem before playing the piece. Ms. Cookie also rehearsed privately with Amy and Cate to build Amy's confidence. Additionally, to prepare Amy for the Q&A session after the performance, Ms. Cookie invited Amy's school buddies one by one to the rehearsals, first Cate, then Sam, and finally James. Amy was able to gradually talk and answer questions in front of all her buddies. It was a great success when Amy performed in front of the whole class, and everyone cheered for her when she was done. Classmates gathered around Amy and poured their questions in, "How long have you played Guzheng?" "Can you play another piece?" "How come Guzheng has so many strings?" Amy answered using an adequate volume.

## Tips and Tricks

- Parents acknowledge the difficulty of trying out new things. Enable the child to participate instead of opting out by providing different options. Rehearse in advance, including every detail of what to do or say. Prepare a backup plan or "escape route" to keep the child's anxiety at bay.

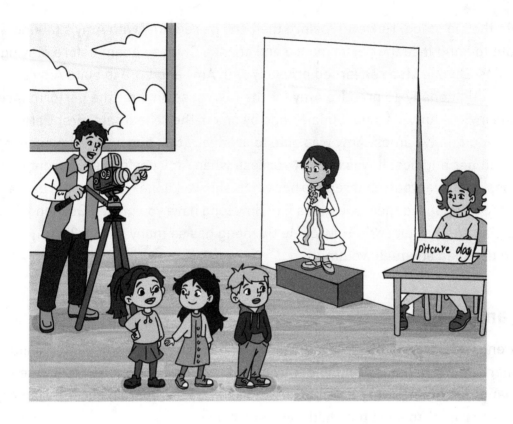

## Picture Day

Today was picture day! Everyone was excited! Even Amy's sloppy classmates who wore their t-shirts inside-out were dressed up neatly with slicked-back hair and shining faces, let alone the girls who liked to dress up. But wait! Only one girl was more worried than happy. That was Amy.

Amy waited nervously and silently in line as other classmates were chatting loudly. Amy was dreading her turn because of the big unusual crowd. She kept counting the number of people in front of her every time the line moved up. "5...4...3...2...1..." It was her turn. "Smile", said the photographer. Amy, however, could not smile. Her face was frozen. She had only one thought in her mind, "Take the picture and let me go". "Say cheese...or you can just show me your beautiful teeth. All right, little mouse? Eek, eek!" The photographer tried to make a light-hearted joke.

Amy could not hold back her giggle at the photographer. The camera flashed, and Amy's smiley face was perfectly captured. Amy jumped down from the stool and beamed with pride.

## Tips and Tricks

- Teachers can introduce the photographer to the child beforehand. The adult can let the child know what will happen on the picture day and help the child rehearse how to take a picture.
- Teacher and the child's buddy can inform the photographer about the child's SM condition, i.e., he/she gets nervous in front of strangers and a big crowd.
- Rather than giving children options to opt-out, offer them choices that are less stressful. For example, the teacher can bring the child to take the picture before everyone else does.

# Part 5

# SUPPORT FOR THE CHILD AT HOME AND IN THE COMMUNITY

This section aims to provide support for children with selective mutism (SM) at home and in the community, highlighting the significance of playdates and child participation in developing connections and relationships with peers. It offers guidance on arranging successful playdates, including recommended activities and strategies to encourage communication.

It is best to organise playdates at home whenever possible to create a comfortable and secure environment. However, community-based playdates can also be beneficial if hosting at home is challenging or not feasible for the child's age. In addition, parents can encourage their child's involvement in group activities such as team sports, small animal clubs, and birthday parties to foster friendships and build confidence and social skills.

This section outlines scenarios that Amy has encountered and draws on her experience to offer tips and advice in different situations.

The section encourages parents to explore different options and activities that align with their child's interests, talents, and specific needs, providing examples that can be adapted based on individual circumstances. The overall goal is to inspire parents to take an active role in facilitating their child's social development and creating opportunities for meaningful interactions with peers.

DOI: 10.4324/9781003355267-5

# Playdate – Essential Component No. 5 in SM Recovery Journey

Complete the Playdates Tracker before each playdate and update it afterwards.

Playdates encourage exposure with fun activities and games that both parties enjoy:

- Multiple exposures with the same person or group of people in a similar location, such as home, friend's home, park, or school playground.
- Well-planned activities can make sure everyone in the playdate has fun.

1. **Parents' role**

   - Lead the support team, including siblings, relatives, teachers, classmates, friends, tutors, nanny, coach, etc. Facilitate communication through games and activities.
   - Parents organise, support, and join games in a playdate.
   - Use recommended strategies to connect the child and classmates.
   - Play video/audio and let the child's voice be heard.

2. **Classmates and friends, number of people attending, situation, and location**

   - Playdate with classmates is the priority, as they will be on the rainbow bridge to connect home and community to the school. Buddy system is dynamic and can be personalised according to each child's condition and situation. During a playdate, parents need to facilitate the conversation. At the beginning of the playdate, children may not communicate. But with the right guidance and strategies, the child may open up and have a talking buddy at the end of the playdate.
   - In the beginning, focus on one or two classmates to have playdates. Through consistent and frequent playdates, these classmates will become the child's talking buddies and maybe best friends, the core components of a buddy system.
   - After the child is used to having regular playdates, invite as many classmates, one at a time, to expand the child's talking circle. If possible, involve a talking buddy to accompany the child in these playdates, further accelerating the progress.

3. **Frequency and length of playdate – The more playdates, the better the progress**

   - To get a better result, three times a week is recommended (this was effective with Amy).
   - Minimum half an hour each time.
   - The day trip, sleepover, vacation, and camping will accelerate the progress.

4. **Offer help to others**

   - Give a ride to the after-school club, help with homework, teach cooking and baking, babysit, and volunteer.

**TABLE 5.1  Playdate five factors facilitating communication**

| No. | Factors in playdates | Examples | | |
|---|---|---|---|---|
| 1 | Playdate should have fun activities/ games for both parties | ❑ Role play at home | ❑ Use pet to connect child and peers in the school playground | ❑ Meet in public places, park, restaurant, zoo, etc. |
| 2 | Parent/sibling leads and facilitates conversation | ❑ Mom at birthday party | ❑ Dad at school garden club | ❑ Siblings at after-school program |
| 3 | Situation: Number of people, what's happening, location, and environment | ❑ Number of classmates and friends | ❑ Types of activities | ❑ Location: Community park |
| 4 | Length and frequency | ❑ Length: Overnight trip is better than a few hours of playdate | ❑ Frequency: Three times a week | ❑ Regularly with the same classmate to foster friendship |
| 5 | Parent offering a helpful hand and convenience to others (car ride, babysitting, volunteer) | ❑ Give classmates a ride to the small animal club | ❑ Teach children how to bake | ❑ Volunteer in non-profit organisations |

**TABLE 5.2  Activity five factors facilitating communication**

| No. | Activity type | Example | | |
|---|---|---|---|---|
| 1 | Non-verbal and verbal communication – gestures, writing, drawing, making sound, talking (start quietly and gradually get louder) | ❏ Role play – cashier | ❏ Use a pet bird as an intermediary and mimic bird's sound | ❏ After school program doing Homework |
| 2 | Movement | ❏ "Marco Polo" game | ❏ "Catch me if you can" | ❏ Release butterflies |
| 3 | Team/group activities without competition. The children are working towards the same goals | ❏ Dance team | ❏ Garden club | ❏ Yard sale |
| 4 | Activities/games with competition | ❏ Play soccer | ❏ Turn-taking game | ❏ Team up to win a game |
| 5 | Fun and exciting | ❏ Camping | ❏ Small animal club | ❏ Jumping on trampoline |

# Form 5.1 Playdate and Progress Tracking

Parents fill out weekly forms to track their child's playdate and progress in communication. Seeing the child's achievements from the tracking sheet motivates parents and children to do more.

The form includes a talking formula (with whom, what, where, situation), a buddy system, and an action analysis. Identify the playmate's relationship with the child and their buddy category: potential, accompanying, talking, and best friends. Note the voice level for a talking buddy with whisper, low, and normal. The goal of the playdate is to foster friendship and move the buddy level up in the system: potential buddy becomes accompanying buddy, accompanying buddy becomes talking buddy, and talking buddy becomes a best friend.

After the playdate, the parents will fill out a playdate analysis section on the form. Write down the strategies used during the playdate, the child's progress, and areas for improvement. The form will serve as both a schedule for the playdate and a self-check for evaluating its success. This will help parents identify effective strategies and areas where they can improve.

| No. | Date | Talking formula | | | | | | | Playdate analysis | | | |
| --- | --- | --- | --- | --- | --- | --- | --- | --- | --- | --- | --- | --- |
| | | Who – Name | Who – Classmates/others | Who – Buddy system | Activity | Location | Situation | Strategies | Progress | Improvement | | |
| 1 | | | | | | | | | | | | |
| 2 | | | | | | | | | | | | |
| 3 | | | | | | | | | | | | |
| 4 | | | | | | | | | | | | |
| 5 | | | | | | | | | | | | |
| 6 | | | | | | | | | | | | |
| 7 | | | | | | | | | | | | |
| 8 | | | | | | | | | | | | |

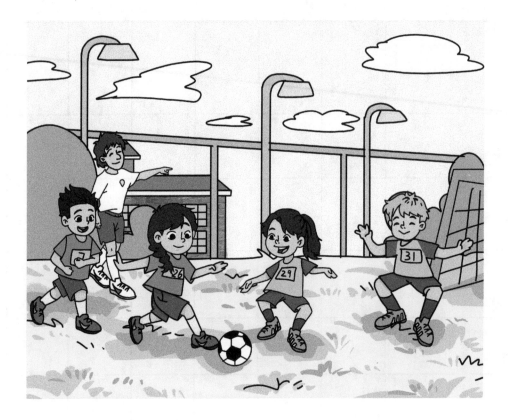

## Team Sports – After-School Program Hosted in School

"Amy! Watch out for Cate!" Amy's soccer teammate, David, called out. Amy heard, turned her body to shield Cate, and looked around. "To me, Amy!" David called out to her. Quick as a flash, Amy kicked the ball to David. Suddenly Amy spotted a gap. "Here, David!" she shouted. Everyone was fully immersed in the game, and no one paid attention that Amy had never spoken to them before.

After the game, the entire soccer team, including the coach and parents, got together for dinner. Amy's parents got to know some other parents and arranged playdates and social outings in the near future.

## Tips and Tricks

- Competitive team sports not only benefit the child's physical health but also promote team-building and provide opportunities for spontaneous communication.
- Children with SM can get so absorbed that they 'forget themselves' and talk. Prepare others for this and advise them not to comment or act surprised. They should simply respond as if the child has always spoken.
- Parents can volunteer as a coach or an assistant coach. It will help them find more opportunities to support their child both on and off the field. Parent involvement will help the child be more confident and willing to join social activities.
- For more one-on-one time and rapport building, parents can invite the coach to a home visit, set up playdates with teammates, and give teammates rides to the practices and matches.

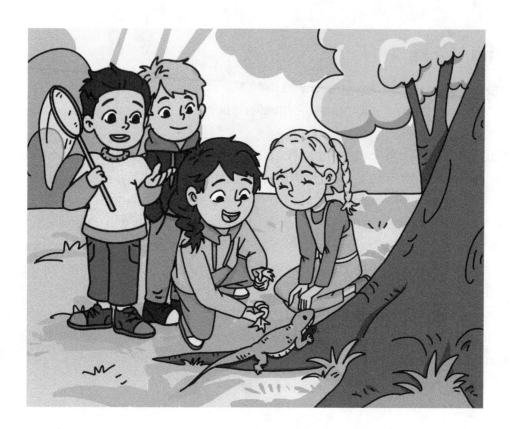

## Small Animal Club

Amy felt relaxed around animals because she knew animals never expected her to talk. Amy joined a small animal club with her classmate Sam. They fed birds, chased ducks, and petted bunnies. Amy had been playing with animals silently until her brother Tom joined the club as a volunteer.

When Tom and Amy saw a lizard climbing on the tree, Amy asked her brother in a whisper, "Tom, can lizards climb really fast?" "Let me ask Sam", Tom replied. "Can lizards climb the tree..." Tom spoke the first part of Amy's question and then looked at Amy. After a short pause, Amy quietly said, "Really fast?" Sam happily answered, "Yes, I think so!" It was the first time that Sam heard Amy's voice. Looking at the lizard, Tom started to take the lead in imitating the sound of a lizard, "hiss". Amy pretended to climb like a lizard while saying "hiss". Then Sam joined them in doing the same thing.

After the club, Amy's mom gave Sam a ride home. Inside the car, the children made all kinds of animal sounds and named different animals. At first, Amy said animal names behind her stuffed animal. Then as she got comfortable, she was able to talk without hiding behind her toy.

## Tips and Tricks

- If speaking words is too difficult for the child in the beginning, try to navigate the child to make different animal sounds instead. For example, start with a simple "Ssss" for a snake sound or "Zzzz" for a bee sound. Then move on to "moo", "meow", and "oink".
- Child joins an after-school club with at least one of their classmates in order to feel more comfortable. Parents or siblings can volunteer at the club and act as a bridge to bring the child's voice into the club.
- Parents should let the club teacher/coach know the dos and don'ts when working with a child with selective mutism.

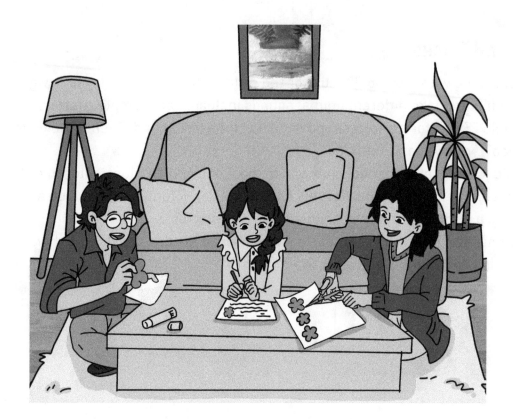

## Birthday Party 1 – Birthday Party Invitation

Amy's birthday was approaching. Amy hand-crafted her birthday party invitations with her parents' help. The invitations included not only information about the date, time, location, and food but also a description of exciting games and activities such as piñatas, face painting, and a magic show.

Amy and her buddy Rosa distributed the invitations to their classmates one by one, "Do you want to go to Amy's birthday party?" Rosa asked their classmates, and Amy handed over the invitations. After asking a few classmates, Amy and Rosa switched roles. "Do you want to come to my birthday party?" Amy asked, and Rosa handed out the invitations instead. The classmates were very excited and asked Amy all kinds of questions, such as, "Are you going to put lots of candies and toys in the pinata?" "Is there going to be a clown or a real magician at the party?" "What do you wish for your birthday present?" Amy was able to answer some questions directly. For other questions, she either spoke softly to Rosa or used her Talking Album that she had prepared in advance.

## Tips and Tricks

- Parents can request from the teacher a list of classmates' names if needed. Use birthday parties, special occasion celebrations, or simple gatherings as a great opportunity to invite as many classmates as possible. It will help the child socialise and expand the circle of friends in addition to sparking conversations in a more casual and fun setting.
- The teacher, the child, and the talking buddy can practise distributing invitations, collecting RSVPs, and discussing birthday preparations in a small group.
- A Talking Album is a book with a recording function. Each page has a pocket for one or two pictures, and the built-in microphone allows you to record a message about the picture.

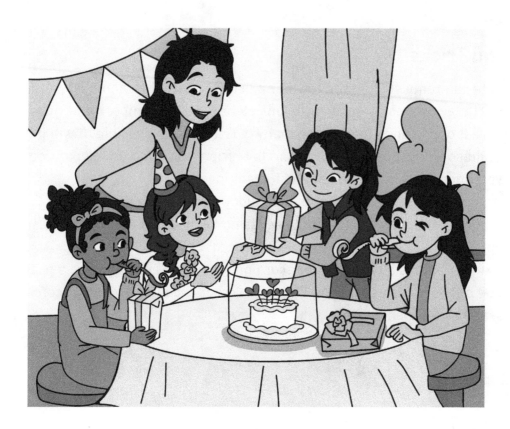

## Birthday Party 2 – Welcome Friends

Amy was up early today to prepare for her birthday party. She reviewed her checklist: face painting table, check; piñata filled with candies, check; magic show, check. Mom was making phone calls to confirm guests were coming. Amy joined the calls and said "thank you" at the end of the conversation.

Amy was happy that her classmates, friends from Girl Scouts, her dance team from the after-school program, and a friend she had known at preschool would all be coming. She might not talk to some of them, but she agreed with Mom to open the door for everyone and say "thank you" when others wished her "Happy Birthday!". An optional message for Amy to deliver was, "Party is over at 5 pm, and pick-up starts at 5:10". Mom agreed to help if Amy got stuck.

Ding, ding, ding! The first guest, Amy's talking buddy and classmate, Sofie, had arrived. Amy jumped up, gave Sofie a big hug, and then went inside to play together. Oh, wait, Amy ran out of the door and yelled to Sofie's mom: "The party will be over at 5 pm. Please pick Sofie up at 5:10". "Sounds good! Happy birthday and have fun!" Sofie's mom laughed.

More friends and parents came. Amy managed to greet them. Sometimes, she spoke at a normal volume; other times, she talked by whispering or just using gestures, depending on how familiar she was with the person. Nonetheless, Amy was having a great time.

The gifts were piled up and looked so pretty. When Amy received the gifts from her friends, she had no trouble saying "Thank you." She even guessed what was in the gift box. Amy's mom was screaming happily inside but pretending nothing special had happened. Mom recorded this exciting moment and shared it with Amy's teacher.

## Tips and Tricks

- Assign the child a job and rehearse in advance. For example, let the child join the confirmation calls to give the child a chance to talk over the phone, and let the child greet guests and make the announcement for pick-up time.
- Hosting a birthday party at home with fun activities will help the child connect to classmates much more easily than in school. The child will feel less anxious in the home environment.

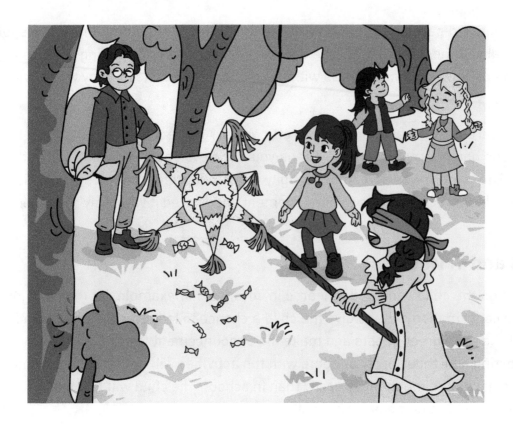

# Birthday Party 3 – Piñata

It was time for piñata! Everyone got together in the backyard and couldn't wait to take turns hitting the piñata. After each child was blindfolded, Amy held his/her hand carefully and led him/her to the piñata. Others started to count, "one, two, three, go!" before the child swung the stick to hit the piñata. Being blindfolded and spun around a few times, it is not easy to walk close to the tree and hit the Piñata. All children laughed and giggled at everyone's wobbly steps, whether they hit the Piñata or not. Amy started to help her classmates by telling them, "the Piñata is right in front of you; move the stick higher, now hit". It took a while for the Piñata to start to crack.

Now it was Amy's turn. She swung the stick with all her strength, and "bang!" candies flew out from the piñata. All the children ran to pick up the colourful candies, counted, and traded them with each other. Amy's mom videoed these memorable moments to share with everyone.

## Tips and Tricks

- Involve the child in the party planning, e.g., making and distributing birthday invitations, shopping for party decorations and foods, etc.
- Ensure the child that there is "no pressure to talk" and always prepare a back-up plan if the original plan does not work out. If the parents of classmates keep asking Amy many questions, if her classmates make a lot of noise and ask Amy to sing with them, and if the magician asks Amy to be an assistant, Amy can ask a talking buddy to help her out.
- Provide positive feedback. Tell the child how well he or she has done, how his or her hard work will pay off, and how proud you are of them.

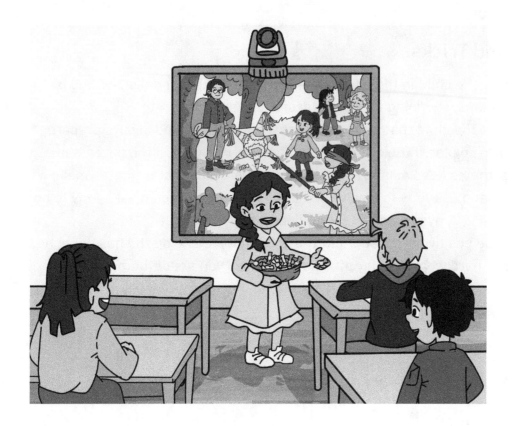

## Birthday Party 4 – Class Presentation of Birthday Party Video

As agreed with her teacher, Amy shared her birthday party video in the classroom and explained to her classmates how to make a piñata. Amy felt at ease showing the video because most of her classmates attended her party. Everyone laughed when the video showed Amy tricked her best friend, Cate, who missed hitting the piñata. Amy smiled and said to Cate, "Sorry, but I brought your favourite candy". Amy took out a basket of colourful candies and passed them out to her classmates.

Next, Amy explained the steps of making a piñata which she had rehearsed several times at home, "First, you blow up a balloon, glue layers and layers of colourful paper on it, and let it sit and dry. After everything is completely dried, pop the balloon, and add a long string to hang up the piñata on the tree. Please don't forget to add yummy candies inside before you hang the piñata". "Amy, I cannot believe you made the piñata at home!" "Yeah, it looked so beautiful!" The classmates praised her work. They continued commenting and asking questions about face painting, the magic show, games, and food. No one realised that Amy had never talked so much and so naturally in front of the whole class before.

## Tips and Tricks

- A well-planned and executed birthday party can be a turning point for a child's communication in school. Showing the child's video to classmates helps the classmates understand what the child is capable of.
- When presenting in front of a class, the child can choose to show a video with their voice recorded. Rehearse the presentation and prepare for Q&As ahead of time. Have a talking buddy standing next to them if additional support is needed.
- Take advantage of the child's interests, talents, and special occasions whenever possible. It will lead to opportunities for the child to stand out and build on confidence.

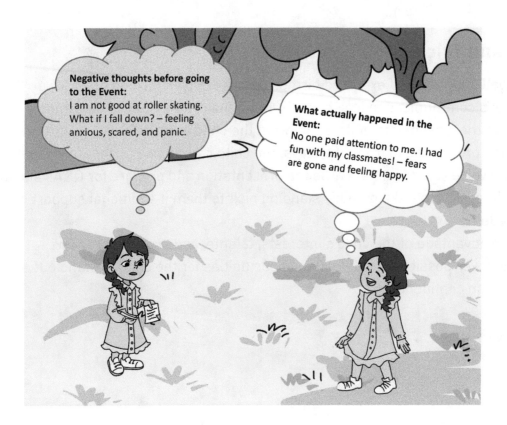

## Negative Thoughts and What Actually Happened

Amy was invited to her classmate's roller-skating birthday party. She wanted to go but was worried about falling and becoming the centre of attention. "I don't want to be stared at by others when I fall. What if they ask me if I am hurt and need help?" Amy told her worries to Mom. "Amy, remember you had a blast at Sam's trampoline party last time? You had the same worries before you went. But everything turned out fine, and you had a fantastic time. How about we go to the party early with your buddy Sam and check out the facility first? If you don't want to roller-skate, you can bring Sam's favourite board game to play with her during her break, or we can leave after half an hour". Amy's mom reminded Amy of her past positive experience and offered a back-up plan. Guess what? It turned out Amy had a great time roller-skating at the party.

## Tips and Tricks

- Suggested support: arrive early to get familiar with the environment and activities; play privately/in a small group before everyone arrives; learn roller-skating before the party; give a ride to a talking buddy, and hang out together at the party.
- Escape Plan: instead of roller-skating, bring a game to play instead, or agree to leave after going around the rink once with mom or a buddy.
- Positive Experience: "I can roller skate!" A positive experience can build the child's confidence and encourage the child to try new things.
- Jot down what happened: The record (example form below) can show a child's progress. The child will see things are not as scary as they thought.
- Practise, Practise, and Practise: Once the child has a positive experience, keep doing it, as it gets easier every time.

## Form 5.2 Recording How the Child's Feelings Change before and after an Activity

(Parents can have examples to discuss with the child when needed.)

| | BEFORE | | | AFTER | |
|---|---|---|---|---|---|
| Date | Negative Thought | Suggested Support | Escape Plan | What Happened | Positive Experience |
| | | | | | |
| | | | | | |

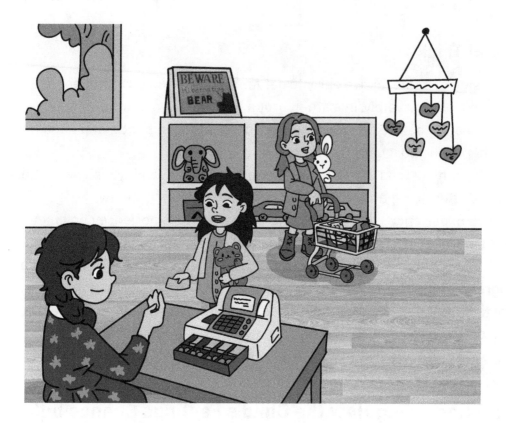

## Playdate at Home – Shopping Role-Play

Today, Amy had a playdate with two of her classmates, Marissa and Rosa. Before they began playing, Amy's mom played a video of Amy's previous playdates. Marissa and Rosa could clearly hear Amy's voice, but their attention was drawn to the fun activities shown in the video. Since no one commented on Amy's voice, Amy did not feel embarrassed.

Then, the girls went on to play one of Amy's favourite games, a shopping role-play. Amy pretended to be a cashier. Marissa was the customer. She walked up to Amy and asked, "How much is this bear?" Amy whispered, "$5". Marissa went on, "Please give me a teacher discount". "Have you got a ID?" Amy asked. "Sure". Marissa showed Amy her "Teacher ID". Amy was feeling generous. "Okay, after the discount, your total is $3", she said. Good thing that I played with my mom before, and she asked for the same discount... Amy thought to herself. Amy and her mom also agreed before the playdate that Amy could help put items on the shelf or put a label on the "shopping goods" if Amy did not want to be a talkative cashier anymore.

## Tips and Tricks

- Playdates are effective in helping children talk to their classmates, especially when they are young.
- Playdate at home makes the child feel relaxed, and parents have more control over the activities. Playdate in a public place, such as a park, gives children more opportunities to play exciting and sporty games. Gradually children will have the confidence to attend playdates at their friends' homes.
- The number of children in the playdate should start with one and increase one at a time. Talking to one classmate is less difficult than speaking in front of a group.
- In a role-play game, children may be more comfortable talking in different roles. Such as acting out being a particular character in a book, cashier in the store, or waiter or waitress in a restaurant; they can also incorporate games with sound, musical instruments, and playing with puppets.

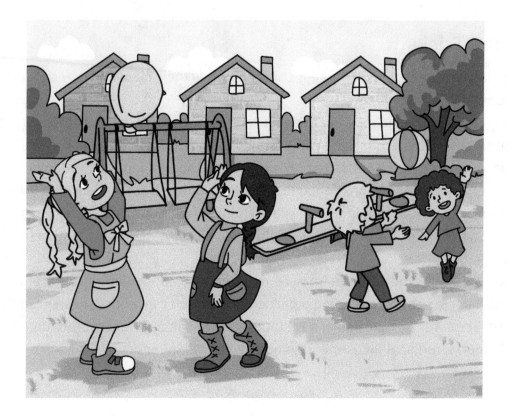

## Playdate in Community

Amy invited her classmate, Sam, for a playdate in the community park. Amy and her mom arrived early to play a balloon-throwing game. Each time they threw a balloon to each other, they would loudly or quietly say a colour, such as "blue, "red", and "yellow". When Sam arrived, she was invited to join the game. Mom and Amy demonstrated how to play the game, then Sam joined in. Now three of them were playing the game. Whenever they threw the balloon into the air, each of them would take turns making an animal sound, "cluck", "meow", "squeak", "moo", "baa", until they ran out of sounds. Mom withdrew from the game after seeing Amy playing comfortably with Sam and watched from the side. Later, Amy's dad came, so Amy and Sam teamed up to compete with Amy's parents. The winners could get a reward of their choice. The two girls were super excited and eager to win the game, so they chose to call out their classmates' names. Sure enough, Mom and Dad ran out of names first!

More neighbours' children came to the community park. Some of them were Amy's classmates. "Can I join you?" they asked Sam, because they knew that Amy had never responded to them before. They knew Amy as a not talking girl. "The balloon is Amy's; you should ask Amy", Sam responded. "Amy, can I play with you?" they asked Amy. Amy either nodded her head or thumbed up. Occasionally, she said "yes" to her buddy.

## Tips and Tricks

- Playing in the community park makes it easier to meet classmates and neighbours.
- The five factors of a good game are language, action/movement, competition, teamwork, and fun/excitement.
- Having a playdate with the same classmate on several occasions is more effective for building rapport than inviting a number of classmates for one playdate.
- A playdate should be long enough for the child to get warmed up and fully engaged in the game.
- Help children accept it when others win the game, e.g., allowing Sam to win.

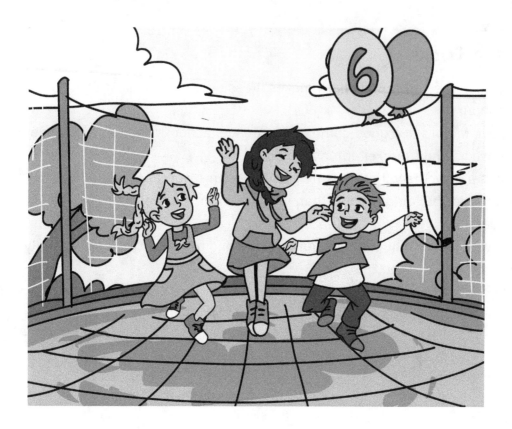

## Attending a Birthday Party

Amy was invited to her best friend Sam's trampoline birthday party. With Mom's help, Amy prepared a "birthday gift survey" to show Sam in school. When Sam marked "hairpin, silly socks, two front teeth..." on the gift list, she and Amy giggled and made silly jokes. Even though Amy was looking forward to seeing her best friend at the birthday party, the unfamiliar crowd made her anxious. She began to worry about what would happen at the party and many "what ifs". Mom tried to cheer her up by reminding her of a positive experience she had at the previous roller-skating party. "Amy, we will arrive early to check out everything before everyone else comes. Let's bring your favourite board game to play with Sam if you don't feel like joining others". Mom reassured Amy.

No one could resist jumping on a trampoline, not even Amy. "Let's play 'tag,'" Sam suggested once they were on the trampoline. "Tag me!" Amy jumped away quickly and smiled at Sam. "It's hard to catch you!" Sam said. "Let's count how many times we can jump and not fall down", Amy called out loudly while a boy joined their jumping. The three of them counted while jumping. Amy was having a great time. By the end of the party, she was already looking forward to another party.

## Tips and Tricks

- A survey gives the child an opportunity to initiate conversation. The survey can cover a range of topics such as favourite festivals, food, pets, and more. The child can work independently or with a talking buddy to distribute and collect the survey forms while teachers and classmates complete the survey questionnaires.
- SM children take longer to warm up in a new setting. Arrive early to get familiarised with the venue first. Parents should facilitate and help the child join group activities. Stay until the end of the party to have more one-on-one time with other children if group activities are too challenging for the child.
- Parents can use the party as an opportunity to meet other parents to build rapport and arrange playdates/attend the same after-school club/program. All of which will help expand the child's circle of friends.
- Parents can ask for a party activity/game list and practise games and activities with the child at home.
- Prepare a plan B, knowing that there is a possible escape route will reduce the child's anxiety and make plan A more likely to succeed. For example, leave after giving the child the birthday card and present, only stay for an hour, or sit with Mom and watch rather than join group activities.

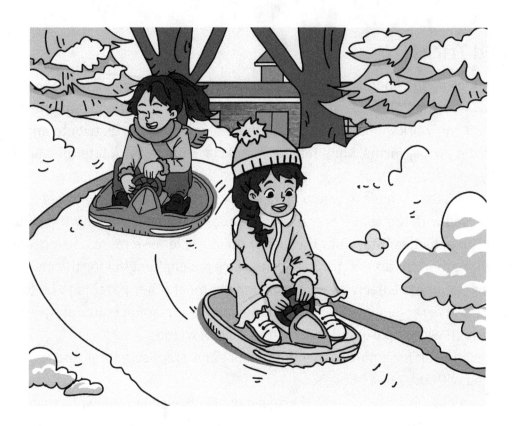

## Go Snow Sledding with Classmates

Amy and Mom came to pick up Cate to go snow sledding. "Amy, I will wait in the car. Please knock on the door and ask for Cate". Mom gave Amy an opportunity to challenge herself. Looking forward to snow sledding with Cate, Amy decided to give it a try. "Can Cate come with me snow sledding?" Amy quietly asked when Cate's mom opened the door. "Of course. Do you want to come in?" Cate's mom asked. "No, thank you, my mom is waiting in the car. We will go to the hill next to the school".

Amy and Cate dragged their snow sleds quickly up the hill. Cate asked excitedly, "Amy, let's see who can slide down faster!" Amy said, "Ok!" "One, two, three, go!" Cate shouted. "Let's do it again!" Amy shouted after they reached the foot of the hill. More and more children came to ride the sled. Cate saw her friend Leah. "Let's play together, Leah!" Cate called out. So the three children rushed to the top of the hill. When it was Amy's turn to count down, she said loudly, "One, two, three, go!"

"Whoo-hoo! Yippee!" the girls yelled exuberantly.

"Goodbye!" Amy said to Leah loud and clear when they parted. On the way home, Amy told Mom that she was invited to Leah's birthday party, and her best friend Rosa would be there too.

## Tips and Tricks

- When the child really wants something, they will be more motivated to take up the challenge. Arrange playdates with exciting activities to boost the chance of verbal communication.
- Children often do more when their parents are not beside them, so do not be afraid to hold back and show children that you have faith in them.
- Set up the next playdate at the same activity with new friends to expand the circle of friends.

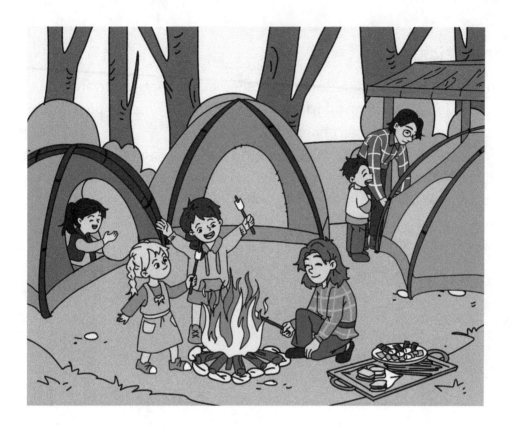

## Camping with Classmates and Neighbours

Amy was excited about her first camping trip. She had always liked nature, which made her feel relaxed and free. She went with her family and a few neighbours and classmates. Everyone went to work once they arrived at the campsite. Some were assigned to help set up the tents and beds. Some were asked to collect stones and wood to start a campfire.

Amy was assigned to the cooking team. She helped fill the trays with crackers, marshmallows, chocolate, and fruits while Sam's mom successfully started a campfire. "Can we start to make S'mores?" Amy asked Sam's mom, even though she had never talked to her before. "Do you know how to make S'mores?" Sam's mom asked, poking the fire without looking at Amy directly. She was pleased that Amy felt comfortable around her. "First, put the marshmallow on to a bamboo stick, roast the marshmallow on fire, then use the top of a graham cracker to move the marshmallow over, add the chocolate, and EAT!" Amy raised her voice at the end, feeling excited.

"Wow, wow, wow, your S'more looks so good! Who made it? Is it tasty? How can you make the marshmallow such a nice shade of brown and not burn it? May I get one?" Sam's dad approached Amy with many questions. Amy's mom and Amy's talking buddy, Sam, did not come to rescue her. They all trusted that Amy could manage the questions. Sure enough, Amy was able to answer and make a beautiful S'more for Sam's dad.

## Tips and Tricks

- It takes longer for SM children to get familiarised in a new setting and be willing to participate in group activities. Parents can plan weekend trips with the child's preferred activities and locations in mind. The goal is to spend extended time with friends, neighbours, classmates, etc., to allow the child to build rapport with them.
- Whether going out or inviting a new child home for a playdate, the potential candidate is best suggested by the child or recommended by the child's teacher. Any adults involved should know about SM and how to approach a child with SM.

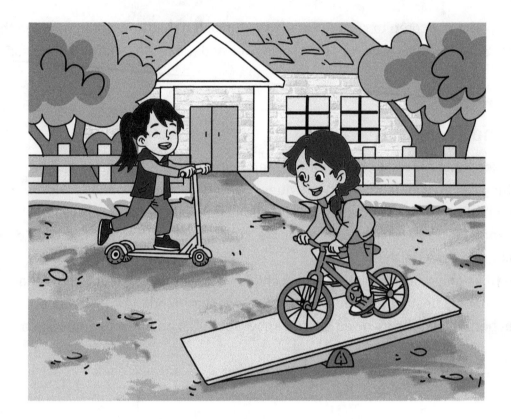

## Talents and Skills – Play with Neighbours in the Community

Though Amy loved to play outside, she did not know how to 'join in' on games or activities. Most of the time, she played alone, watched her neighbours play, or simply stayed home. Amy's parents found that neighbours' children loved to play card games/board games/table hockey, ride on bikes/scooters, jump rope, and even play ping-pong. Soon, Amy got all kinds of new gear to practise and became good at them.

Amy and her parents started a game in the corner of the playground. The neighbours' children came over to check out what they were playing. Amy's parents facilitated her in showing (non-verbal) or telling (verbal) the rules of the game. Once Amy engaged with other children, her parents slid out.

"Amy, do you want to come out to play?" from that day on, Amy received more and more invitations from her neighbours. Amy ran out with her new bike and chased her friend Jada who rode a scooter on the street. Later, they met more neighbours on skateboards and roller-skates. Amy learned the bike skill of jumping on boards and speeding down hills, which made her very proud since she had just recently learned to ride a bike.

## Tips and Tricks

- SM children are slow to warm up to people outside their comfort zone. Parents will need to play alongside the child and create opportunities for other children to join their games/activities.
- Parents stay with the child to facilitate interactions and only leave when the child is fully engaged and able to communicate either verbally or non-verbally.

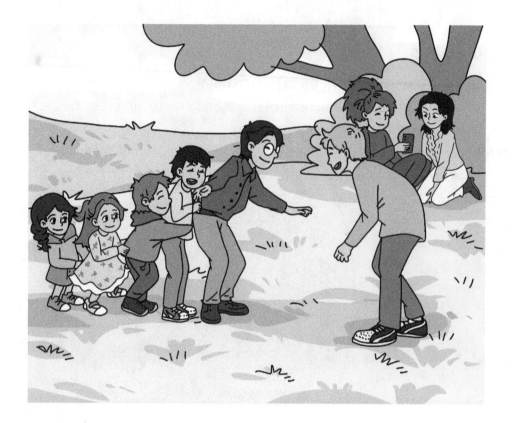

## Catch Me If You Can – Fun Time with Families and Friends

Amy's family was hanging out with their cousins and friends in the park. Kids were playing with dads for a "Catch me" game. Amy's dad was the protector of all the little ones. Dad's best friend, Uncle Michael, was the attacker who tried to catch the child at the end of the line. They were running, chasing, and screaming. Both adults and children were having a great time.

Amy's mom and Aunt Waiyee sat nearby, watching the video of Amy's yard sale. They kept commenting and laughing. "Amy, come over". Mom invited Amy to watch the video together. "Were they your neighbours or classmates? Who made lemonade for you, Mom or Dad? How much did you charge for a cute teddy bear?" Aunt Waiyee asked graded questions and waited for a few seconds to let Amy prepare her answers.

## Tips and Tricks

- Parents prepare a supporter name list consisting of family members, cousins, friends, and neighbours. Peers who are close in age are preferred. Build rapport by having a small group gathering at home/in the park, travelling together, visiting friend's home, and doing sleepovers. Playdates are more effective when occurred consistently and frequently with the same child/family for an extended period.
- Parents inform supporters about the child's challenges and provide basic knowledge of SM. Before two families/children get together, they can send each other voice recordings/videos, listen to recordings of silly noises, watch videos, or facetime.

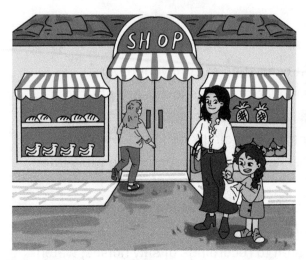 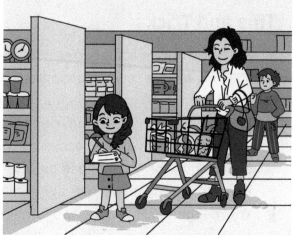

## Shopping 1 – Discuss the Shopping List before Arriving (Left) and Check off the Items on the Shopping List (Right)

One of Amy's favourite pretend plays on her playdates was shopping in the supermarket. She could quickly get into her role and interact with her friends using words. They learned the names of various foods and practised the shopping routine. As a shopper, Amy searched for items on her shopping list. When she could not find something, she would ask her friend, who pretended to be a salesperson. "Where can I find potato chips?" Amy asked. "In aisle 3". her friend answered. After they finished shopping, Amy switched from being a shopper to a cashier because she was good at maths. "Your total came up to be $49.99. Would you like to pay by cash or card?" Amy asked while pretending to operate the register.

Mom's best friend, Aunt Linda, promised to take Amy shopping in the supermarket. They prepared a shopping list together in advance. Linda asked Amy to draw pictures next to the words "bread, watermelon, pineapple, sprinkles, milk, and cheese" on the list. These visual reminders helped build Amy's confidence in communication. Before entering the supermarket, Linda and Amy went over the list and discussed who would pick up which items. Amy chose her favourite items on the list: cheese and sprinkles! Amy went back and forth in the supermarket for her items and asked Linda to confirm if she had picked the right item before checking it off the list.

Retrieving the shopping items with Linda helped build Amy's confidence and made her feel like a "big girl".

## Tips and Tricks

- Children often talk more in a supermarket than in a small grocery store which might be very quiet; others can hear the child and might stand too close to him or her.
- The shopping list should be attractive and exciting for the child. Discussing the recipes and how to cook the meal with the child so he or she is eager to shop.
- Rehearse the shopping process at home and before going to the store. The practice helps prepare the child, so he or she knows what to do or say in different scenarios. Role play game is one of the best ways for a young child to rehearse the scenarios.
- Bringing a talking buddy with the child could make the shopping experience fun, and the child is more likely to have a dialogue.

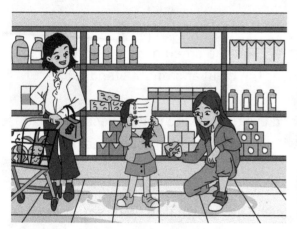 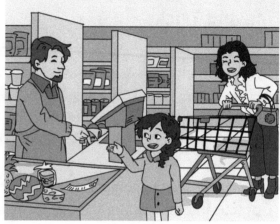

## Shopping 2 – Get Help from the Clerk without Speaking (Left) and Check Out Items and Pay at the Cashier (Right)

Linda was busy picking up items from the shelf near Amy. "Linda, I can't find the cheese anywhere", said Amy. "Please ask a clerk", Linda replied. When a clerk passed by, Amy put her shopping list on her face to get the clerk's attention. It was a smart move! The clerk noticed Amy and looked at the shopping list. She took the cheese from the shelf and showed it to Amy, "Is this the right one?" Amy removed the list from her face and nodded. "Is it for macaroni cheese or a hamburger?" the friendly clerk guessed. "Macaroni", Amy answered in a low voice while looking at Linda. The clerk told Amy how much she loved macaroni and cheese. "Do you need anything else?" The clerk must have realised that some items on the shopping list were not marked off yet. "Sprinkles", Amy answered in a voice louder than before.

At the checkout, Linda gave Amy an opportunity to communicate with the cashier by standing behind Amy and keeping a little distance from the cashier. "Do you need any bags?" asked the cashier. Linda waited this was one of the things they'd practised during role-play at home. "Do we need bags, Amy?" she repeated. "No, thank you!" Amy said to the cashier and continued unloading the shopping cart. "Did he say

$36.55?" Linda asked Amy, pretending that she hadn't heard. "No, $26.55", Amy repeated the amount to Linda in front of the cashier. "Card or cash?" asked the cashier. Again, Linda waited. "Card or cash?" called out Amy loudly. "Oh, sorry", Linda laughed, "I was miles away! Cash, please".

## Tips and Tricks

- The child is more willing to try something new and challenging if he or she is motivated. Shopping for items they are interested in helps to boost their willingness to take on the challenge. Non-verbal communication, e.g., taking items from the clerk and handing the money to the cashier, help the child build confidence prior to verbal communication.
- Before the child takes on challenging work like asking for the price or location of specific items, parent or other accompanying adult should begin a casual conversation with him/her and make sure that the child talks to the parent or adult in front of the shoppers and clerks (or other strangers)
- In a relaxed environment, the child is more likely to communicate with a soft-spoken clerk who does not expect the child to respond. The positive shopping experience will encourage the child to do more and take one step (or a few steps) forward.

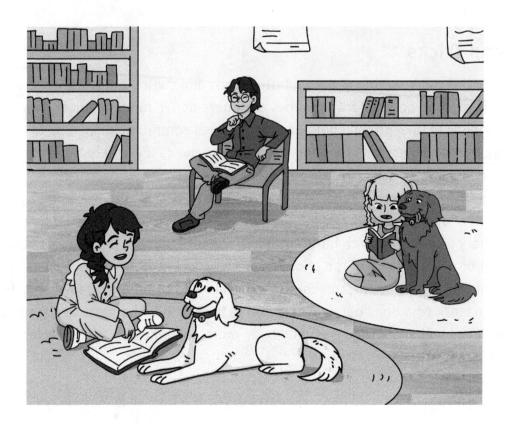

## Reading Paws in Township Library

Amy and her talking buddy Sam were going to the town library to attend an event called "Reading Paws". Some service dogs would be there to keep readers company. Amy and Sam got excited when they saw many cute dogs in the library. Sam went to a brown puppy and read next to him.

Amy loved the Reading Paws program, where one could read to a service dog or just sit and listen to others reading books; there was no expectation to talk.

Last time, she came with a friend and listened to her reading. Today, with Dad, Amy walked into the library and saw a milky white puppy sitting quietly on the carpet. When the dog owner asked Amy if she would like to read to her dog, Amy nodded. The dog owner then asked, "Which book are you going to read to my princess?" Amy picked a book and started to read, "A long, long time ago, there was a pretty little girl named Katie..." Amy read slowly and softly, page after page. Her voice got louder and louder as she read on.

After reading one book, Dad told the dog owner that Amy had a question for her. "May I pet 'Little Lady'?" Amy asked shyly. The dog owner kindly replied, "Of course. But how do you know her name?" Amy smiled and pointed to the dog's name tag. While Amy was playing with Little Lady, she started to talk to the dog. She completely forgot that the library was full of strangers.

## Tips and Tricks

- Let the child know ahead of time who are the safe strangers they can talk to. Instead of talking directly to strangers, help the child to talk in strangers' presence first. Do not pressure the child to talk if it is too difficult at the moment. Simply praise them for what they have accomplished and encourage them to try again at another time.
- Rehearse the conversations at home to prepare the child for talking to strangers in public. For example, what they need to say to a cashier at the check-out or how to ask a librarian to find a book of their interest. The child can choose to memorise, pre-record their messages, or read off from a script.
- Choose a setting where the child is more motivated to talk to strangers, for example at an ice cream shop or a petting zoo.
- Reading aloud is a good way to help children get their first words out if they read well it is more predictable than conversation, so it creates less anxiety.

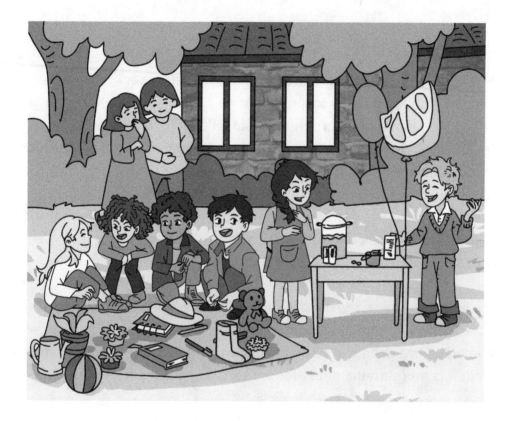

## Yard Sale and Lemonade Stand in the Community

Amy's cousins and neighbours were holding a yard sale with a lemonade stand in the community. Amy was invited to join and asked to be the cashier since she was good at maths. Amy's cousins did all the talking. Amy helped out wherever needed, e.g., setting up the lemonade stand, showing the customers of their interested items, collecting payments, etc. Amy had fun at the yard sale with her cousins and neighbours. Even though she did not talk much, the positive experience made her want to join more group activities later.

## Tips and Tricks

- Building a buddy system both in and outside of school with classmates are the two sides of the Supporting Triangle. Most of the activities in this book are related to these two sides.
- A third aspect of the Supporting Triangle involves creating a buddy system between home and the community, involving neighbours, friends, cousins, and children of the parent's friend or coworker. Playdates with individuals from this third aspect can be conveniently arranged and scheduled as frequently as desired, whether on a daily basis, a few times per week, or weekly.
- Sometimes, talking to a stranger (the third aspect) may be easier than talking to familiar people who expect the child to talk on a regular basis. Engaging in activities such as yard sales, lemonade stands, and shopping in the market offers opportunities to practise interacting with strangers.

# Part 6

# OVERCOMING SELECTIVE MUTISM AND GAINING SOCIAL SKILLS

This section is intended for older children currently dealing with selective mutism (SM) and those who have recently overcome it. For teenagers with SM, the most effective strategy we found with Amy was to seek opportunities to meet with peers, friends, and strangers of all ages. Joining clubs or sports teams, volunteering, and working part-time jobs are excellent ways to engage in social activities and enhance communication skills. For children who have recently overcome SM, it is crucial to maintain the momentum gained from starting to speak and continue developing their social and communication skills, as these skills will prove beneficial throughout their lifetime.

DOI: 10.4324/9781003355267-6

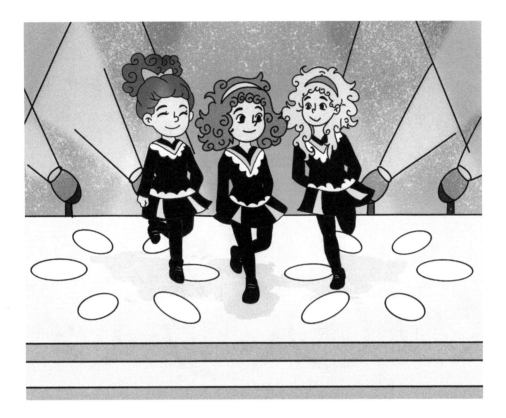

## Dance All the Way – Amy Overcomes SM

Dancing, joining clubs, and doing volunteer work had accompanied Amy along her SM journey. It had helped her build confidence and friendship, allowed her to attend competitions, and participate in community performances/services. Being a Girl Scout helped Amy make a circle of friends who grew up together and supported each other. All the events, trips, camping, and volunteer works that Girl Scouts did together created a strong bond among themselves. Amy received much help from her buddies; in return, she helped others whenever she could. Conquering her challenges one at a time made Amy who she is today – smart, caring, and unstoppable!

When a child can talk anytime, anywhere, with anyone, they can proudly say that they have overcome SM! It is no longer challenging for them to present in front of a large group of unfamiliar people, share opinions, praise others, initiate social interaction, and meet new people.

However, parents need to know that it takes time to build the social skills the child missed in their SM years. Some children with SM are naturally on the quiet side, but most are not. Though they might NOT be social butterflies, they are NOT a child with SM anymore. The child has come a long way in learning to respond to questions from non-verbal to sounds, words, phrases, and sentences, from passively answering questions to asking questions and initiating conversations. With SM years behind them, the child can now embark on a new journey with their full potential.

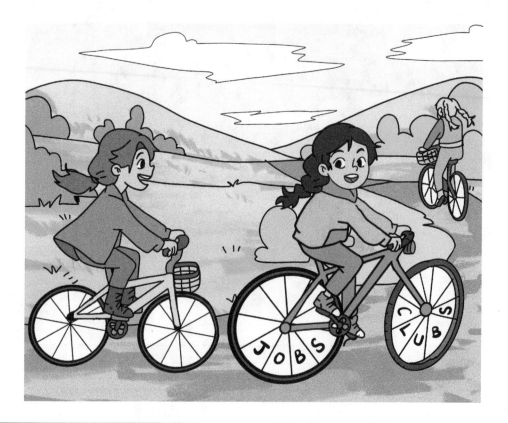

**Back Wheel – Jobs (Paid or Unpaid)**

1. Camp counsellor
2. Supermarket cashier
3. Restaurant waiter/waitress/host
4. Babysitter
5. Pet sitter/walker
6. Tutor
7. After-school program helper

**Front Wheel – Clubs/Teams**

1. Drama club
2. Debate team
3. Boy/Girl Scouts
4. Sports team
5. Service club
6. Animal shelter helper group
7. Science club

## Going Out and Moving Forward – Gaining Social Skills through Clubs, Volunteering, and Jobs

Even though a playdate is highly effective in building rapport with peers, forming a buddy system, and expanding the circle of friends, when the child gets older, such as a teenager, it is not so easy to invite peers home for a playdate. However, the young person can go out to meet other children with the same interests through various activities, such as clubs, sports, volunteering, and part-time jobs. These activities will provide unlimited talking and social opportunities.

Going out to meet others also helps the child who has overcome SM move forward, as he/she still needs time to rebuild social skills. When Amy is spending time with friends in clubs, reading a book to the preschool children, being a stage manager supporting a theatre production, walking a dog on the street, selling candles in the market..., she is moving forward to build a social and fulfilling life.

Every child is unique. We hope parents get inspired by these examples and develop social activities based on the child's interests, abilities, personalities, and other qualities that fit their specific situation.

# INDEX

Page numbers in bold indicate tables, and page numbers in italics indicate figures.

after-school clubs 49–52, 124–26, 182, 184–85, 220–21; animal sounds 13, 134, 184–85, 198

anxiety 33, 200; and classroom placement 158–59; and the five factors 14; hand chart for 16, 130, 132; and negative thoughts 194–95; others' reactions 171; and school 53; school layout schema 132; and subject helper roles 151–52; tests 166

art 106, 162–63

bathrooms 2, 4, 11, 19, 26, 54, 139–40

best friends 25, 26–27

birthday parties 186–87, 188–89, 190–91, 192–94, 194–95, 200–01

buddy system 9–10, 11–12, 17, 19, 25, 26, 30, 32, 177, 217; bathroom buddies 26, 139–40; breaks/recess 141–42; classmates 9–10, 23, 24, 26, 39, 53, 122, 170; and daily routines 39, 54, 131; expanding 111; forms 27; friends as 10, 23, 24; school bus 39, 53, 55–56; sliding in 57; talking buddies 12, 26, 30–31, 38, 51, 64, 77, 86, 88, 90, 108, 110, 113, 122, 157, 160, 162, 180, 191, 211

bullying 170–71

butterfly project 143–45, 147–50

camping 204–05

children: opportunities for 17, 19; staying involved 35–36

children with selective mutism: building social skills 219–21; characteristics of xx, 166; easier locations in classrooms 158–59; encouraging 37; involving in action plans 39; strengths recognition for 130, 172; volunteering by 50

class assignments 122, 156; answering questions 63, 154, 157; non-verbal participation 158; rehearsing 77, 112–13, 147–48, 172–73; tests 166–67

class presentations 112–13, 147–48, 193

classmates: and birthday parties 186–89; buddy system 9–10, 23, 24, 26, 39, 53, 122, 170, 177, 217; playdates with 177, 202; and summer connections 128; and teacher's helper roles 120

commentary style talking 60–61, 96–97, 106–07

communication activity five factors 179

communication books 43, 77, 79, 113, 116–17, 165; task books 118, 119

communication stages 13, 30, 155

community parks 198–99, 206, 208

confidence-building 17, 36, 45, 71, 193, 210, 219

conversations, rehearsing 30–31, 36, 56

cookies 92, 96, 98

daily routines, and the buddy system 39

desensitisation 81, 107

dos/don'ts: for parents 33–34; for teachers 81–83

empathy 155

essential eight components 17, 18

essential management trio 17, 21

extracurricular classes 124–25

five factors communication activity 179; playdates 178; talking 14

5-second rule 63, 77, 122, 154, 157, 164

forced choice questions 13, 31

forms: anxiety hand chart 16, 130; negative feelings 195; playdate tracking 180; rewards 44; task books 119; teacher's helper 153

4W and 1H 22

games-playing 19, 28, 31, 32, 36, 47, 58, 60, 62, 64, 66, 68, 70–71, 86, 90, 93, 108, 114, 126, 128, 135, 141–42, 179–80, 198, 206 see also small-group play

gardening club 49

Girl Scouts 51–52, 219

goal-setting, and rewards 42, 43, 45

graded exposure 107

graded question sequences 38, 61, 76–77, 89, 91, 114, 134, 157, 208

greeting students 135–36

group activities 176 see also after-school clubs; extracurricular classes

helper name list form 24

Individualised Education Plans (IEPs) 31, 78, 90

jobs 220–21

jokes 104–05

kayaking 35

libraries 157, 214–15

Montessori philosophy xx

music classes 158, 172–73

negative reinforcement cycle 8

negative thoughts 194–95, 200

neighbors 204, 206

new people, introducing 60–70

nonverbal communication 13, 54, 77, 136, 167, 171, 212; and rewards 42

one-on-one 18–19, 22–23, 67, 73, 75, 79, 82, 105–07, 114–15, 142, 146, 183, 201

others: help from 10; in the SMart Village 23, 24

parental support 9, 17, 18, 28, 32, 50, 201; after-school activities 49–52, 127; communication books 116–17;

dos/don'ts 32–33; in the essential management trio 18, 21; and the 5-second rule 63, 77; helper name list form 24; importance of 30–31, 36; letters to teachers 76–77; morning routines 133–34; and new people 60–65, 69, 206–07; and playdates 177, 178, 196–97; at school 18, 28, 32, 48, 58; shopping 211, 213; in the SMart Village 23; tracking 28, 119, 153, 180, volunteering 28, 30, 32, 47–48, 51–52, 59, 183
part-time employment 220–21
parties: birthday parties 186–87, 188–89, 190–91, 192–94, 194–95, 200–01; holiday parties 168–69
patience 77
passing over taking over 13, 63
perfectionism 166
pets 37–38, 42, 133–34, 137, 150, 178, 214
piñatas 186, 188, 190, 192
playdates 12, 17, 19, 33, 47, 127, 176–77, 178–79, 180–81, 196–99, 202–03, 209–10, 217, 220; five factors 178
pre-recording messages 49, 55, 113, 154–55, 167, 215 see also videos; voice recording toys
preschool 2
private tutors 124

questions 154, 157, 164; encouraging answers 37–38, 48; forced choice 31; graded question sequences 38, 61, 76–77, 89, 91, 114, 134, 157; from other kids 39

rainbow bridge 12, 25, 177
rapport-building 63, 69, 73–74, 91, 100, 105, 111, 114, 121–23, 127, 205, 220
reading aloud 156, 214
Reading Paws program 214–15
recovery journey 9, 10
Reitman, Amy, experiences of xxiv, 2, 35
rewards 40–41, 42, 45, 46, 119; forms 43–44
rewards calendar/system 40–41, 42; forms 43–44; goal-setting 42, 43, 45, 46; long-term vs. short term 42–43
role-play games 196–97, 210–11

school: Back to School Night 86; breaks/recess 141–42; cafeteria 18, 28, 32, 47–48, 54, 104; counsellor's office 66, 68, 70, 90, 145; grades 166; group-working 110–11; gym class 142, 160–61; holiday parties 168–69; keyworkers at 117; missed assignments 166–67; morning routines 133, 137; moving up grades 88; as overwhelming to SM children 47–48; parents volunteering at 28, 30, 32, 47–49; picture day 174–75; playgrounds 37–38; playing games at 58; SM impacts on 4, 6; summer breaks 100–01, 128–29; support systems at 31, 66–67, 69–71, 85, 155; talent shows 172–73; teacher introductions 60–65; visiting 84–85, 88, 129; washrooms 2, 11, 19, 26, 54, 139–40
school bus 39, 53, 55–56
school challenges, identifying 131
school layout schema 131, 132
second languages 124
The Selective Mutism Resource Manual 2nd Ed (Johnson and Wintgens) xxii
selective mutism (SM) xxiii, 2–3; as anxiety disorder 2–3, 33, 76; experiences of xxiv; helpful insights

about 5; misconceptions about 5; physical symptoms 4; school-related symptoms 4; social/emotional symptoms 4; support guidance 1; talking about 170–71
The Selective Mutism Workbook for Parents and Professionals (Reitman and Johnson) xx, xxii
self-education 71, 159
self-modelling 107
shopping 210–13
sledding 202
sliding in strategy 57, 97
SM treating professionals (SMTPs) 17, 18, 20, 20–21, 30; helper name list form 24
small animal club 185
small-group play 110, 114, 126, 160, 178–79, 196–97
small steps 29, 31–32, 43–46, 71, 73
SMart village 17, 19, 22, 23; helper form 24
social impacts of SM 4, 6
Spanish language classes 124
sports 160, 182
sportscaster communication 60–61
strangers 217
subject helpers 151–53
success, experiencing 40–41
summer breaks 100–01, 128
supermarkets 210–11
supporting triangle 11, 217
surveys 201

talking albums 186–87
talking birds 49
talking bridges 59, 65, 67, 69, 74, 85, 87, 99, 125, 127, 133
talking circle 102, 177; expanding 39 see also buddy system
talking five factors 14
talking formula 14, 179
teachers 73, 125; helper name list form 24; home visits 18, 32, 74, 92–98, 103, 122; introducing 60–65; as keyworkers 99, 117; lack of support from 7; one-on-one time with 60–65, 74, 106–08, 114, 122, 146; outside of school 102; parental letters to 76–77; as part of the team 17, 18, 21, 78; school cafeteria 104; shadow teachers 74, 122–23; shadowing 121; in the SMart Village 23, 24; substitutes 164–65; in the summer 100–01; supportive behaviors from 7, 9, 76–77, 79–81
teacher's helpers 120, 131, 137, 151–53, 158, 162
tips/tricks/recommendations 3, 7, 15; after-school activities 52, 125, 127, 185; animal sounds 134, 185; answering questions 157; art 163; Back to School Night 86; breaks/recess 142; buddy system 54, 56, 87, 148, 163, 211, 217; camping 205; class assignments 113, 144; classmates 217; communicating needs 167; communication books 113, 117, 165; community parks 199; escape routes/plan 148, 173, 195, 201; extracurricular classes 125; first arrive last leave 87 games-play 36, 63, 69, 71, 91, 93, 97, 107, 109, 111, 199; graded question sequences 38, 61, 71, 91, 99, 107, 134, 155, 157; greetings 136; gym class 161; introducing new people 61, 63, 65, 71, 73; jokes 106; morning routines 138; negative feelings 195;

new experiences 173; nonverbal communication 136, 167, 171, 213; one-on-one with teachers 107, 109, 115, 146; parental letters 77; parental support 31, 36, 50, 59, 127, 134, 201, 207, 213, 215; parties 170, 187, 189, 191, 193, 201; pets 134, 150, 201; picture day 176; playdates 38, 59, 87, 127, 129, 171, 183, 197, 199, 203, 209, 217; practise 30, 56, 59, 71, 105, 140, 144, 146, 150, 167, 187, 195, 201, 217 rapport-building 101, 105, 111, 123, 146, 205; reading aloud 215; rehearsing 148, 152, 173, 193, 211, 215; rewards system 40, 41, 46; role play games 211; school support systems 67, 71, 85; school visits 85, 87, 89, 129; shadow teachers 123; shopping 211, 213; sports 183; strangers 217; subject helper roles 152; substitute teachers 165; summer breaks 129; surveys 201; talking about SM 171; talking albums 187; teacher home visits 93, 95, 97, 99, 103; teacher support 155, 159, 175; teacher's helper 121, 138; teachers outside of classes 103, 105, 115; tests 167; voice recordings 91, 95, 101, 107, 109, 144, 146, 209, 215; volunteering 49, 183, 185
toys, talking through 54
turn-taking 69, 114

verbal communication: indirect 13; initiating 13; pre-recorded 49, 55, 113, 154–55, 158, 167, 215; responding 13; and rewards 42
videos 47, 66–67, 76, 84, 98, 101, 107, 112, 114, 125, 143–44, 158, 189–90, 192–93, 208–09
voice exposure 74, 90, 94–95, 107, 146 see also videos; desensitisation
voice messages 100–01
voice-recording toys 49, 54, 135
volunteering: by parents 28, 30, 32, 47–49, 51–52, 59, 182; by SM children 50, 219

whispering 26

yard sales 216

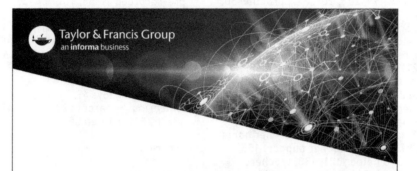

Printed in the USA
CPSIA information can be obtained
at www.ICGtesting.com
LVHW071449171223
766686LV00022B/1658